Common Pitfalls in Multiple Sclerosis and CNS Demyelinating Diseases

Case-Based Learning

Common Pitfalls in Multiple Sclerosis and CNS Demyelinating Diseases

Case-Based Learning

B. Mark Keegan
Mayo Clinic College of Medicine, Rochester, MN, USA

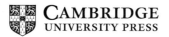

CAMBRIDGE
UNIVERSITY PRESS

University Printing House, Cambridge CB2 8BS, United Kingdom

Cambridge University Press is part of the University of Cambridge.

It furthers the University's mission by disseminating knowledge in the pursuit of education, learning and research at the highest international levels of excellence.

www.cambridge.org
Information on this title: www.cambridge.org/9781107680401

First published 2016

Printed in the United Kingdom by TJ International Ltd. Padstow Cornwall

A catalogue record for this publication is available from the British Library

Library of Congress Cataloguing in Publication data
Keegan, B. Mark, author.
Common pitfalls in multiple sclerosis and CNS demyelinating diseases :
case-based learning / B. Mark Keegan.
Cambridge, U.K. ; New York : Cambridge University Press, 2016. |
Includes bibliographical references and index.
LCCN 2015042977 | ISBN 9781107680401 (paperback)
| MESH: Multiple Sclerosis – diagnosis – Case Reports. | Multiple
Sclerosis – therapy – Case Reports. | Demyelinating
Diseases – diagnosis – Case Reports.
LCC RC377 | NLM WL 360 | DDC 616.8/34–dc23
LC record available at http://lccn.loc.gov/2015042977

ISBN 978-1-107-68040-1 Paperback

Contents

Preface

This book is a case-based instructional that will assist the reader in evaluating patients with neurological presentations that may be due to central nervous system demyelination, particularly multiple sclerosis (MS), and distinguishing the presentation of MS from other competing neurological diagnoses. This book is of importance for a number of reasons. Some people have neurological symptoms and signs that are due to MS. It is critical to make a confident MS diagnosis, particularly given the new, expanding and broadening availability of therapies for relapsing forms of MS. Just as importantly, however, many people have neurological symptoms and signs that are not due to MS, and have an alternative neurological diagnosis or, in fact, no neurological diagnosis or disease. It remains just as critical to provide a diagnosis and therapies for "other" neurological diseases where available, or guide the patient away from potentially toxic therapies for a suspected MS that is not present.

The book is aimed at those with some degree of neurological education and experience; however, a highly structured approach to MS diagnosis, namely a three-step diagnostic process, is emphasized throughout to demonstrate how even complicated presentations may be "made simple" to ease the evaluation. Initial chapters explain this diagnostic process and how it is used to diagnose MS. Subsequent chapters proceed on an anatomical basis to evaluate MS presentations in that level of the central nervous system and MS-mimicking diseases that constitute alternative diagnoses. The chapters are presented in anatomical order to assist the reader if they come across a challenging case with a certain anatomical presentation by providing direct references to potential MS mimickers at different levels of the nervous system.

Diagnosing neurological diseases is easier when a structured diagnostic process is used and when prior experience has provided other examples where "pattern recognition" facilitates rapid identification of a certain disease. This book therefore provides a three-step process to help the reader diagnose MS in patients.

The cases themselves are selected to present decision-making points using the three-step process to assess how likely or unlikely the presentation represents MS. Key diagnostic and therapeutic tips are provided to highlight the main points regarding each case. Comprehensive and detailed discussions about the pathophysiology and treatment of MS and mimicking diseases are not emphasized and the reader is directed to further references that will provide a more exhaustive level of detail.

It is hoped that this book, with its highly clinically relevant cases and straightforward manner of assessing challenging presentations of MS and related diseases, will be an enjoyable and informative addition to standard textbooks of these conditions.

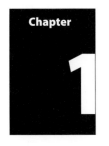

Pitfalls in identifying the classical clinical features of MS

Introduction

Multiple sclerosis (MS) is the prototypical inflammatory demyelinating disease of the central nervous system (CNS). While it is the most common presentation of this spectrum of diseases, other inflammatory, infectious, structural, genetic disease processes and even normal presentations are competing diagnoses. While in the past it was difficult in some cases to make a clear diagnosis of MS based mostly on clinical evaluation, current investigational technologies, particularly brain and spinal cord magnetic resonance imaging (MRI), have made this far easier today. It is critical to make a confident and definitive diagnosis of MS prior to administering effective MS medications in order to avoid potentially toxic therapies aimed at different disease processes. In this introductory chapter we approach a simplified three-step assessment when diagnosing MS:

Three-step diagnosis of MS

Step 1: Identify the classical clinical features of MS
Step 2: Conduct a neurological examination for signs of MS
Step 3: Assess investigational evidence of MS

Step 1: Identify the classical clinical features of MS

See Table 1.1.

One way to diagnose multiple sclerosis with confidence, as opposed to competing diagnoses, that will be encouraged in this book is to undertake a three-step diagnostic evaluation. The first step involves identifying the presence or absence of the classical, clinical features of multiple sclerosis. This includes, but is not limited to, optic neuritis, diplopia, trigeminal neuralgia, dysarthria, ataxia, hemiparesis, hemisensory loss, Lhermitte symptom and symptoms

of acute or progressive myelopathy (sensory level, paraparesis or quadriparesis, sphincteric dysfunction). Apart from paroxysmal symptoms of MS, such as trigeminal neuralgia and painful tonic spasms, which are discussed further in Chapter 3, most symptoms that are classified as new clinical attacks of multiple sclerosis should last at least twenty-four hours but usually last days to weeks in duration. For instance, a common presenting symptom of multiple sclerosis is optic neuritis. The typical history in a patient with optic neuritis is of painful, unilateral, central visual loss that worsens over hours to days. The visual loss may plateau over a number of days to weeks and then improve spontaneously or with the use of corticosteroids, again over many weeks. Visual improvement often may be excellent but recovery may be incomplete. Painless loss of vision is less common a manifestation of optic neuritis due to MS, as is binocular loss of vision. These latter findings should prompt a careful search for an alternative cause for the visual impairment.

In contradistinction to the painful nature of optic neuritis, diplopia due to MS should be painless. This condition should also be "binocular" in nature, in that if the patient closes one eye, the diplopia is abolished as the visual input is coming solely from the uncovered eye. It may be vertical or horizontal or oblique in nature. Diplopia of most etiologies comes on acutely, but the severity of the diplopia due to a demyelinating cause may worsen over hours to days.

MS patients may develop Lhermitte symptoms. This is an unusual paresthesia of a "shock-like" or "buzzing" sensation that occurs classically on extreme neck flexion. This is indicative of a demyelination within the cervical spine and is produced by the neck flexion stretching the spinal cord, which leads to demyelinated axons being hyperirritable and discharging unnaturally with this stimulus. This symptom, while characteristic of MS, may also occur in patients with other causes of cervical myelopathy

Table 1.1

Symptom	Classical clinical features	Pitfall symptoms
Optic neuritis	Painful, monocular visual loss	Painless, binocular loss, refractive error, migrainous visual auras
Diplopia	Painless, binocular, long duration	Monocular, brief duration (seconds to minutes)
Trigeminal neuralgia	Lancinating shock-like pain with typical triggers (e.g. touching, speaking, cold air)	Constant facial pain
Sensory symptoms	Sensory level (spinal cord level); hemisensory impairment (cortical/subcortical level); alternating sensory loss ipsilateral face and contralateral limb (brainstem level)	Random, fleeting sensory disturbance in non-neurological distributions
Lhermitte symptom	Shock or buzz on neck flexion	Cracking, popping on neck rotation
Bladder/bowel impairment	Urge-related incontinence	Urinary frequency, anatomical explanations (e.g. pregnancy, surgeries)
Motor and gait impairment	Weakness, or ataxia, often asymmetrical; assess functional limitation; no. of blocks walked, stairs climbed	Restricted activity due to fatigue, pain or deconditioning

such as compressive cervical spondylotic myelopathy and subacute combined degeneration of the spinal cord due to B12 deficiency.

Hemiparesis or hemisensory deficit involving the face, arm, and leg could reflect CNS demyelination within the cerebral white matter. Again, the clues to CNS demyelination as an etiology are the onset and worsening over hours to days, lasting for days to weeks and then improving spontaneously or with corticosteroid treatment. Importantly, symptoms of a sensory myelopathy are common in multiple sclerosis, and this is generally heralded by an ascending sensory level and may be accompanied by quadriparesis or paraparesis (depending on cervical or thoracic location of the lesion) and bowel and bladder dysfunction.

Gait impairment is common in multiple sclerosis, and it is important on a clinical evaluation to identify the actual functional limitations experienced and the exact reasons behind it. For example, many patients have limitations that are due entirely to fatigue or deconditioning. While this limitation is restricting and very important, more compelling evidence of a progressive myelopathy is a reliable onset of

impairing symptoms with less exertion. To use a common clinical example indicative of a progressive myelopathic gait disorder, a patient may describe walking for two miles three years previously, followed by leg dragging at one mile two years ago, then at half a mile one year ago and is now dragging after only walking one city block. If the gait limitation is due solely to ataxia, the number and frequency of falls and requirement of gait aids (walking stick, furniture, other people) constitutes a key informative history. Multiple sclerosis–related gait disorders are generally due to corticospinal track impairment with progressive dragging of one limb or significant gait unsteadiness with falls. Bowel and bladder dysfunction may occur with multiple sclerosis, particularly with lesions of the spinal cord, and may herald as urinary or bowel urgency with associated urge-related incontinence. This should be distinguished from stress urinary incontinence symptoms (e.g. incontinence with coughing, Valsalva strain or laughing) that are often due to anatomical impairment rather than CNS disease.

MS is commonly associated with sensory loss. By far the most sensitive clinical finding of sensory loss due to MS is loss of distal vibratory sense in the

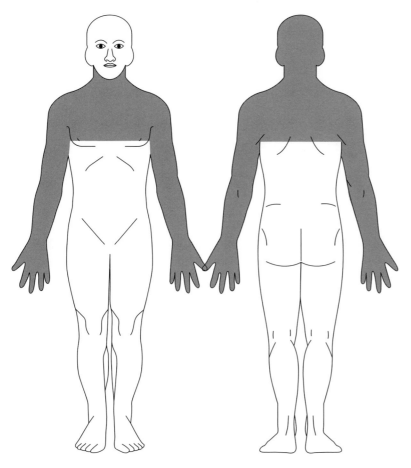

Figure 1.1 Sensory level described by patients with myelopathies.

feet. It should be noted that a "sensory level" indication of a spinal cord impairment, as demonstrated in Figure 1.1, is best evaluated based on clinical history rather than findings on neurological examination. For example, the patient may inform the clinician of a sensory-level pattern. On examination the clinician may or may not be able to identify or confirm the abnormal signs reflecting this impairment, but the clinical history of a definite sensory level should be taken as a highly compelling indication of a spinal cord lesion. An important distinction should be made between a spinal cord sensory level and "large fiber" peripheral neuropathies which may cause similar distal loss of vibratory sense. The clinician should be concerned about a spinal cord lesion when the hands are involved prior to or simultaneously with the feet, and of course if saddle (genital and buttock) region numbness is prominent or if there are signs of upper motor neuron motor impairment consistent with CNS (not peripheral nervous system [PNS]) disease.

Step 2: Conduct a neurological examination for signs of MS

See Table 1.2.

The second step in diagnosing multiple sclerosis, following a detailed evaluation for the classical clinical symptoms of MS, is a comprehensive neurological examination. One way to simplify the results of neurological evaluation is to classify it as normal neurological examination, neurological examination consistent with multiple sclerosis or neurological examination consistent with an alternative neurological disease as the etiology. It should be strongly emphasized that many MS patients will have an entirely normal neurological examination. A neurological examination consistent with MS means that they exhibit one or more characteristic, but not defining or pathognomonic, abnormalities. For instance, patients may have signs of optic neuropathy such as visual acuity impairment, central scotoma, color vision impairment and a pale optic disc,

Table 1.2

Examination	Examination findings	Comment
Dementia	Impaired cognition on mental status exam	Pitfall: non-specific memory concerns are common in MS but not reliably distinguishing; severe dementia is uncommon but occurs in MS
Optic neuropathy	Scotoma, acuity deficit, color vison impairment, relative afferent pupillary deficit	Pitfall: acuity deficit due to refractive errors
Internuclear ophthalmoplegia (INO)	May be bilateral, often incomplete with slowed adduction and dysconjugate nystagmus	Rapid saccades back and forth from extreme horizontal gaze identifies INO
Limb ataxia	Often asymmetrical	Pitfall: palatal myoclonus is a feature of stroke and Alexander disease
Upper motor neuron weakness	Pyramidal distribution; extensor plantar responses (Babinski signs)	Bilateral extensor plantar responses strongly suggest a myelopathy
Sensory loss	In pattern of cortical, brainstem or spinal cord impairment	Distal lower extremity vibratory loss most sensitive; pitfall: pin, light touch sensation is highly subjective and better appreciated on clinical history rather than findings on examination
Gait	Spastic, ataxic quality is most common, often asymmetrical	Pitfall: some patients have functional non-neurological gait disorders, or are impaired by pain

all of which are characteristic of MS, particularly if the patient has a clinical history of typical optic neuritis. Extraocular movement abnormalities such as unilateral or bilateral internuclear ophthalmoplegia (INO) indicative of interruption of the brainstem medial longitudinal fasciculus connecting the oculomotor and contralateral abducens nerve are classically caused by MS. It should be noted, however, that INO due to MS is often incomplete and the identification of slowed adduction with dysconjugate nystagmus is best seen by having the patient make repeated, rapid saccades back and forth from one extreme horizontal gaze to the other. Findings of corticospinal tract impairment with upper motor neuron–type weakness (hyperreflexia, "pyramidal" distribution weakness, extensor plantar responses [Babinski signs]) are commonly found in MS. MS patients may also have signs of cerebellar dysfunction with gait and limb ataxia as well as a cerebellar dysarthria. Distal upper or lower extremity sensory loss particularly to vibration is characteristic of dorsal spinal cord dysfunction in MS.

Step 3: Assess investigational evidence of MS

The third step in diagnosing MS is evaluating the results of appropriately selected investigations (Table 1.3). The most sensitive way to investigate a possible diagnosis of MS is the use of magnetic resonance imaging (MRI) of the brain, cervical, and thoracic spinal cord. Typical ovoid T2-weighted hyperintense lesions located periventricularly within the brain, within the posterior fossa, juxtacortically, chronic T1-weighted hypointense lesions ("black holes") and acute T1 lesions that enhance following gadolinium administration are particularly characteristic of multiple sclerosis (see Figure 1.2). Similar areas of ovoid abnormal T2 signals that are short in length and generally laterally placed are found within the cervical and thoracic spinal cord (Figure 1.3). While it is extremely common to find non-specific MRI lesions within the brain, such as those related to aging, migraine headaches, hypertension and other vascular risk factors, these types of typical T2 lesions within the cervical and thoracic spine are characteristic of multiple sclerosis and do not arise simply due to these conditions.

Table 1.3 Investigational evidence of MS.

- Brain MRI
- Cervical and thoracic spinal cord MRI
- CSF examination: IgG index, unique CSF oligoclonal bands
- Evoked potentials: visual, somatosensory, rarely brainstem auditory evoked potentials
- Serological evaluations for MS mimickers
- Additional evaluations for MS mimickers

The cerebrospinal fluid (CSF) examination remains an important diagnostic test in the evaluation of MS. In particular, CSF elevations in the immunoglobulin G (IgG) index and unique CSF oligoclonal bands are characteristic of an immune-mediated CNS disease process generally and often of multiple sclerosis specifically. Examination of the white blood cell count, protein levels and other values are of benefit, but generally only to rule out mimickers of multiple sclerosis, including CNS infectious diseases, CNS neoplasms or other non-MS CNS diseases.

Electrophysiological evaluation of CNS pathways with evoked potentials also assists in MS diagnosis. Visual evoked potentials (VEP) assess for conduction deficit in the optic nerves. Somatosensory evoked potentials (SSEP) may identify impaired conduction

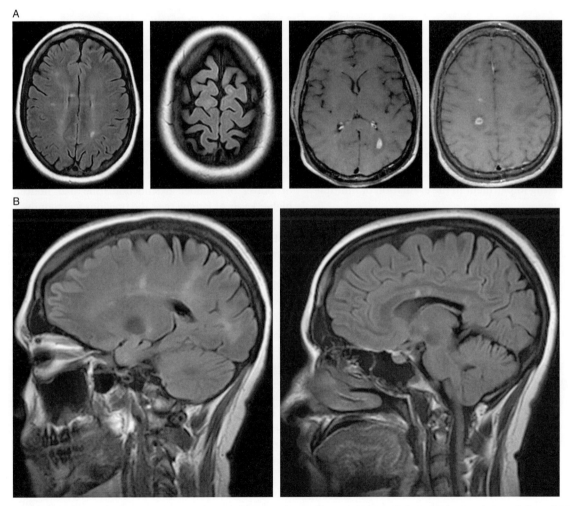

Figure 1.2 A) Axial MRI brain showing typical FLAIR periventricular, juxtacortical and T1 gadolinium–enhancing lesions. B) Sagittal MRI brain FLAIR sequence showing typical "Dawson's fingers" and corpus callosum MS lesions.

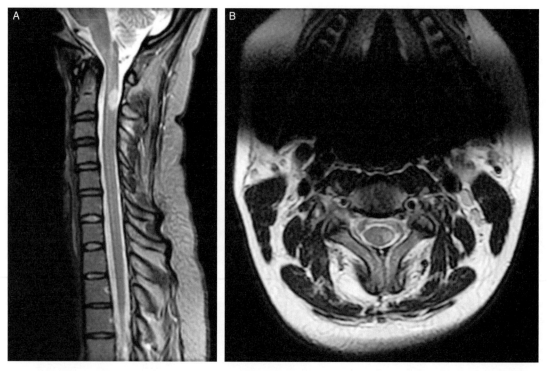

Figure 1.3 Sagittal T2 MRI cervical spine dorsally placed, short-segment, ovoid lesion characteristic of multiple sclerosis. Axial T2 MRI cervical spine in the same patient shows the lesion is in the left lateral aspect of the spinal cord.

in the central proprioceptive pathways. Brainstem auditory evoked potentials (BAEP) may, in rare cases, be useful in identifying central versus peripheral hearing impairment in the evaluation of multiple sclerosis.

Serological and neuroradiological testing, as well as other selected investigations searching for infectious, vascular, traumatic, neoplastic, inherited and other causes that may mimic multiple sclerosis, may be required in cases where a diagnosis of MS remains uncertain (see Table 1.4). Many MS cases are straightforward and few if any investigations outside of MRI, CSF and evoked potentials are required.

Case 1: A woman with numbness and prior visual loss: possible MS

A 41-year-old woman noted one day while showering and shaving her legs that her right leg and thigh sensation was gone. This involved the whole limb, both anterior and posterior. The sensory loss then progressed the next day to involve the foot of that lower extremity, her buttocks, her genitalia, and the next day up to the lower back, all on the right side. She then had

moderate, but incomplete, spontaneous improvement in the sensation over roughly the next three weeks. She had no left-side impairment, nor any motor weakness or bowel or bladder dysfunction. She had noticed higher levels of fatigue over the previous few months.

She recalled that five years previously, during a stressful time, she had left eye blurriness with mild ocular pain that resolved spontaneously over about three or four weeks. She had had no diplopia, dysarthria, dysphagia or hearing loss and no other episodes of visual or sensory impairment. Her ambulation was normal and she could easily walk a mile and recently was able to cycle thirteen miles.

On examination, her mental status was normal, while visual acuity and color vision were normal bilaterally. Her motor exam was normal. A sensory exam revealed decreased temperature sensation up to T5 on the right side, with preserved pin vibratory and joint position sense. Muscle stretch reflexes were normal and her plantar responses were downgoing bilaterally. Her gait was normal.

A brain MRI demonstrated areas of radially oriented nonenhancing increased T2 signals within the cerebral hemispheres, and T2 lesions in the cerebellum and pons suggestive of MS. Gadolinium-

Table 1.4 Clinical and laboratory red flags

Clinical red flags	Implication
Headache/meningismus	Sarcoidosis, SLE, Lymphomatosis
Stroke-like events	SLE, Antiphospholipid Syndrome, CNS angiitis, embolic strokes
Myopathy	Mitochondrial disease, Sarcoidosis
Neuropathy	B12 deficiency, Dysmyelinating D/o
Diabetes insipidus	Sarcoidosis, Histiocytosis
Bone lesions	Histiocytosis/Erdheim Chester disease
Pulmonary symptoms	Sarcoidosis, SLE
Cardiac symptoms	Embolic cerebral infarcts
Mucosal ulcers	Behçet's disease
Arthritis/arthralgia	SLE, Sjögren's disease
Rash	SLE, Fabry's disease, Lyme
Oculomasticatory myorhythmia	CNS Whipple
Uveitis	Behçet's disease, SLE
Prominent family history	CADASIL, Hereditary Spastic Paraparesis, Dysmyelinating disorder
Endocrinopathy	Sarcoidosis, Histiocytosis
Retinopathy	Mitochondrial disease, Susac syndrome
Thrombotic events	Antiphospholipid Syndrome, SLE
Laboratory red flags	
Elevated ESR	Vasculitis, SLE, Sjögren's
High titer ANA	Connective tissue disease
Elevated serum lactate	Mitochondrial disease
Anemia/cytopenia	SLE, B12 deficiency
Persistent/marked CSF pleocytosis	Lymphoma
Neutrophilic CSF pleocytosis	Behçet's disease, CNS Whipple

SLE – systemic lupus erythematosus, CADASIL – cerebral autosomal dominant arteriopathy with subcortical infarcts and leukoencephalopathy

enhancing lesions were found throughout, raising suspicions of active demyelinating disease (Figure 1.4). A cervical spine MRI was normal. A thoracic spine MRI showed subtle, short segment T2–signal abnormality at T4 (not shown). A CSF examination showed elevations in oligoclonal bands and IgG index and normal other values. Visual evoked potential showed mild slowing on the left visual pathway.

Three-step assessment

1 Classical clinical features of MS: sensory myelopathy with resolution, monocular visual loss with pain typical of optic neuritis
2 Neurological examination: myelopathic sensory level
3 Investigations: MRI brain consistent with MS, MRI cervical spine normal, thoracic spine consistent

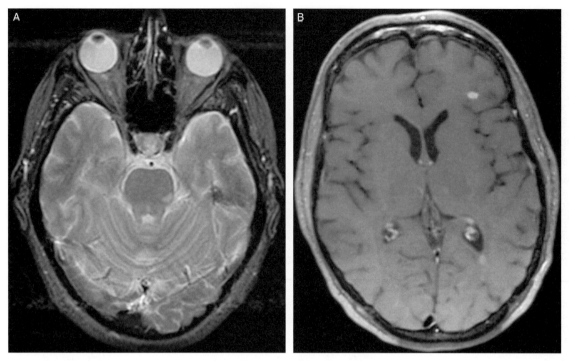

Figure 1.4 A) Axial T2 MRI brain showing left pontine MS lesion. B) Axial T1 MRI brain with gadolinium showing enhancing white matter lesion in left frontal lobe.

with MS; CSF consistent with MS; visual evoked potentials abnormal on left

Diagnosis: Relapsing remitting multiple sclerosis.

Tip: Using the three-step assessment, this patient satisfies all of the steps. She has had classical symptoms of MS attacks with spontaneous resolution including a sensory myelopathy and optic neuritis; her neurological examination is consistent with MS with a thoracic spinal cord sensory level. Important investigations including the brain and spinal cord MRI, CSF examination and evoked potentials are all consistent with MS as the correct diagnosis.

The patient initiated treatment with interferon beta -1a subcutaneous injections three times weekly for relapsing remitting MS.

Case 2: A woman with diffuse pain and abnormal brain MRI scan. It is MS?

A 44-year-old woman presented for evaluation of possible MS. She had a long history of typical migraine headaches without aura, and brain neuroimaging was performed to evaluate the headaches. She described typical migraines with severe headaches that worsened with activity and were associated with photophobia, phonophobia and nausea and vomiting. She had a history of multiple foot surgeries with significant allodynia and complex regional pain syndrome. More recently, she developed more diffuse pain symptoms and it was suspected that she had fibromyalgia. She had symptoms of non-specific memory concerns. Despite this, she was able to prepare all of her meals, go shopping independently and drive without difficulty.

While she had no classical clinical attacks of multiple sclerosis, she reported rare, random, brief, slurring dysarthria as well as word-finding difficulties, but no clear history of aphasia, paraphasic errors, or prolonged dysarthria. She did not have significant dysphagia but occasionally reported rare choking episodes. She had tinnitus but no significant hearing loss. She had a "cracking" sensation on neck movement but no typical Lhermitte symptom (also known as Lhermitte sign). She was limited to walking only one block, but this was entirely due to pain; and she would hold on to her husband because of this.

On neurological examination, she was anxious and appeared depressed but formal mental status

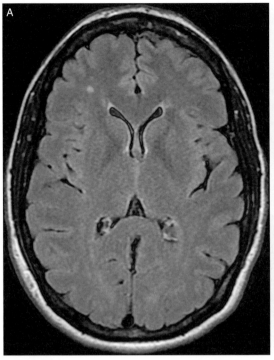
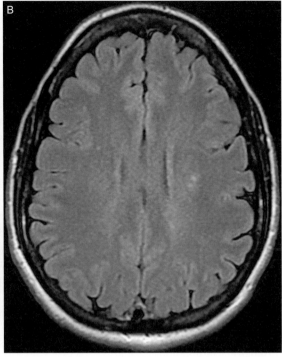

Figure 1.5 Axial FLAIR MRI brain showing commonly found, non-specific, randomly placed signal change, not highly suggestive of MS lesions.

testing was normal. She had an antalgic gait but the rest of her neurological examination was normal.

A brain MRI showed small, non-specific areas of abnormal T2 signal (Figure 1.5). A cervical and thoracic spine MRI was normal and negative for radiological features of demyelinating disease. Visual and somatosensory evoked potentials were both normal. A CSF examination was normal with no elevation in CSF oligoclonal bands or IgG index.

Three-step assessment

1 Classical clinical features of MS: none
2 Neurological examination: normal
3 Investigations: MRI brain: non-specific findings; MRI cervical and thoracic spine negative; CSF normal; evoked potentials negative

Diagnosis: Migraine without aura, fibromyalgia and complex regional pain syndrome, abnormal brain MRI scan with non-specific findings likely related to migraine.

Tip: Diffuse pain, while perhaps common in MS, is not a highly specific, clinically discriminating feature of multiple sclerosis and needs to be investigated thoroughly for alternative causes, such as fibromyalgia.

Complex regional pain syndrome can be the cause of severe focal pain disorders. Undertaking further investigational studies to try to confirm further MS-related abnormalities on spinal cord MRI, evoked potentials and CSF examination is often important to evaluate an abnormal brain MRI with non-specific findings such as in this case.

Case 3: A patient with numbness of the feet rapidly involving the hands. Where is the lesion in the nervous system?

A 43-year-old woman was wrapping holiday gifts when she developed bilateral foot numbness. The next day she noticed similar numbness, now involving the hands bilaterally, and following that had ascending loss of sensation in both lower extremities. The numbness then progressed up the lower extremities to the upper thighs and lower abdomen including the genital and buttocks region, and finally it involved the costal margin. She had no motor weakness or bowel or bladder incontinence despite the lack of perineal sensation. She had no accompanying symptoms of cranial nerve dysfunction and no prior significant symptoms. She had no family history of multiple sclerosis.

On neurological examination, her mental status was normal. Her motor exam was normal throughout, muscle-stretch reflexes were brisk, but plantar responses were flexor bilaterally. Vibratory and joint position senses were normal. Her ambulation was normal.

Brain MRI showed one non-specific area of abnormal T2 signal but was otherwise normal. A cervical spine MRI showed a short segment, oval area of abnormal T2 signal with subtle gadolinium enhancement within the cervical cord at C2 consistent with an inflammatory demyelinating lesion (Figure 1.6). A thoracic spine MRI was normal. The lumbar spine MRI scan was normal with no abnormality of the cauda equina nerve roots.

Three-step assessment

1 Classical clinical features of MS: inflammatory cervical myelopathy
2 Neurological examination: normal

3 Investigations: MRI brain: non-specific findings; MRI cervical spine: typical MS lesion; MRI thoracic and lumbar spine negative

Diagnosis: Clinically isolated syndrome (CIS) of demyelination with inflammatory cervical myelopathy. This is within a relatively low-risk group for future development of multiple sclerosis given the lack of other inflammatory demyelinating lesions compared to CIS patients with >2 asymptomatic non-enhancing T2 MS lesions.

Tip: A sensory "glove" distribution coming immediately following or coinciding with "stocking" distribution should suggest the cervical spinal cord as the level of the nervous system involved. It should not as strongly suggest a peripheral nerve distribution which, if length-dependent and symmetrical, would affect the feet and progressively much travel further up the lower extremities prior to hand involvement ("stocking", then "glove" distribution). A sensory level as was described in the patient above is a symptom that is typically obtained on a clinical history rather than as a clinical finding on neurological examination.

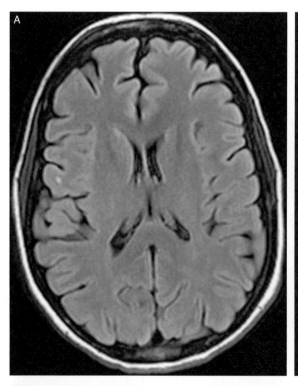
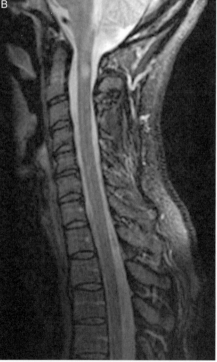

Figure 1.6 A) Axial FLARI MRI brain showing small, non-specific lesion in right hemispheric white matter. B) Sagittal T2 MRI cervical spine short-segment, ovoid lesion characteristic of multiple sclerosis.

Conversely, a sensory level described on clinical history may not be discovered as an abnormal neurological sign despite careful neurological examination but does strongly suggest the presence of a spinal cord disease.

A lumbar spine MRI is not needed specifically in the evaluation of multiple sclerosis per se as a thoracic spinal cord MRI scan shows the entire conus medullaris region to good effect but occasionally can be useful in ruling out a competing lumbosacral radicular cause. In this case, while the cervical spinal cord should be the expected site of neurological symptoms, this test ruled out cauda equina syndrome as the cause of the saddle region anesthesia.

The clinical courses of multiple sclerosis are described in Chapter 2 but in patients with clinically isolated syndromes the MRI may evaluate low- versus high-risk clinically isolated syndromes and inform decision making for clinically isolated syndrome treatment. Those with two or more MS lesions apart from the symptomatic lesion are considered at higher risk of developing MS in the future. High-risk patients may be offered immunomodulatory MS medications for this reason. For those patients with one or no lesions apart from the symptomatic lesion, a "watchful-waiting" approach would be appropriate as they are considered at low risk of developing MS in the future.

Case 4: A patient with a diagnosis of MS presents with new left arm numbness. Is it due to the patient's MS?

When encountering patients with a prior MS diagnosis it should be stressed that new neurological symptoms should not always be presumed to be due to MS. Another way of putting this is that having MS is not protective against other neurological conditions that could present apart from MS. In addition to that caveat, the original diagnosis of MS should continue to be reconsidered and reevaluated in patients to ensure with subsequent evaluations it remains a valid diagnosis.

A 45-year-old woman presented with neck pain and occasional left hand and left-triceps-region paresthesias. She was evaluated twelve years earlier for possible MS where brain MRI lesions were found. She had never had optic neuritis or any other cranial nerve symptoms. She did not have symptoms of ataxia. She had a 15-pack-year history of cigarette smoking and

hypertension for ten years. She had a past history of migraine headaches and a family history of migraine headaches. A second paternal cousin was known to have multiple sclerosis. She was treated with interferon beta preparations intramuscularly once weekly and subcutaneously three times weekly, both of which caused elevated liver enzymes. She initiated glatiramer acetate but had injection site reactions. She was not on immunomodulatory medications for the last ten years.

On neurological examination, her mental status was entirely normal. A cranial nerve examination was normal. Color vision was normal. A motor exam was normal. Her reflexes were normal, and plantar responses were flexor bilaterally. Her gait was normal as was tandem walking. Her sensory exam was normal. Tinel's sign was minimally positive at the left wrist but negative at the right wrist. Phalen's test was negative bilaterally.

A brain MRI showed that areas of T2 signal abnormality had progressed over time, but they were more suggestive of non-specific small vessel ischemic changes rather than MS (Figure 1.7 A). There were no gadolinium-enhancing lesions and no juxtacortical or posterior fossa T2 abnormalities. A cervical spine MRI showed evidence of spondylotic degenerative changes of disc disease which had worsened over time but there were no intramedullary spinal cord signal changes consistent with multiple sclerosis (Figure 1.7 B). A CSF examination was normal without elevations in the IgG index or oligoclonal bands. Evoked potentials were negative for impaired central conduction. Electromyography (EMG) showed evidence of bilateral median neuropathies at the wrist and a chronic active left C7 radiculopathy.

Three-step assessment
1 Classical clinical features of MS: none
2 Neurological examination: consistent with alternative neurological disease – carpal tunnel syndrome, cervical radiculopathy
3 Investigations: MRI brain: non-specific changes; negative CSF normal; EP negative; alternative cause found on electromyography – median neuropathies at the wrist and left c7 radiculopathy

Diagnosis: Median neuropathies at the wrist (carpal tunnel syndrome) and left C7 radiculopathy. No convincing evidence of multiple sclerosis.

Tip: A prior diagnosis of multiple sclerosis should never be assumed even if a patient has been on long-

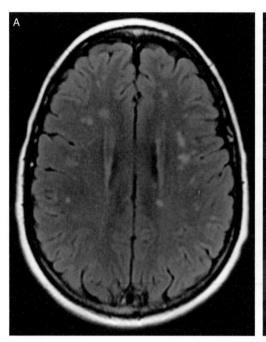
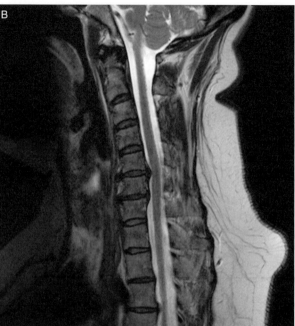

Figure 1.7 A): Axial FLAIR MRI showing brain areas of T2 signal abnormality more suggestive of non-specific small vessel ischemic changes rather than MS. B) Sagittal T2 MRI cervical spine with no changes of MS; disc osteophyte complex at C5 interspace level with mild distortion of the surface of cervical cord without intramedullary signal change within the cord.

term MS immunomodulatory therapy. Reevaluation of a diagnosis of multiple sclerosis regularly is important. Peripheral nerve disease can mimic the sensory and motor symptoms of multiple sclerosis.

Case 5: A young woman with sudden deafness and abnormal brain MRI. Is it MS?

One caveat in assessing patients presumed to have multiple sclerosis is attributing all impairments, no matter how atypical, as likely due to MS. It should be kept in mind that patients with multiple sclerosis may have other causes for neurological impairment, and the diagnosis itself of multiple sclerosis should continue to be reevaluated when new symptoms occur. Some neurological impairment is rarely due to multiple sclerosis and the presence of such neurological symptoms needs to call into question the diagnosis of multiple sclerosis and requires identification of other neurological causes of the presentation.

A 43-year-old woman underwent a brain MRI scan for migraine headaches seven years prior to presentation. It was felt to be abnormal. She sought help

with numerous neurologists and the question arose of whether it was multiple sclerosis. Although initial investigations were inconclusive, she started MS immunomodulatory medications, first with glatiramer acetate and later with interferon beta -1a three times weekly, both of which were discontinued because of intolerable side effects.

She had no prior symptoms suggestive of optic neuritis, diplopia, dysarthria or dysphagia. She had never experienced a Lhermitte symptom nor episodes of hemiparesis, hemisensory deficit or symptoms of sensory myelopathy with resolution. She had a remote history of acute inflammatory demyelinating polyneuropathy (AIDP; Guillain-Barre syndrome) in the past. She had a strong family history of migraine headaches but no family history of MS. One year prior to presentation, she had a sudden onset of deafness involving the left ear. It did not recover, and no other explanation was found for this.

A repeat brain MRI showed multiple areas of nonspecific abnormal T2 signal (Figure 1.8). Cervical and thoracic spine MRI scans showed no evidence of MS. A CSF examination showed oligoclonal bands present in the cerebrospinal fluid; however, all the CSF oligoclonal bands were also present in the serum, indicating a normal result. Somatosensory and visual evoked

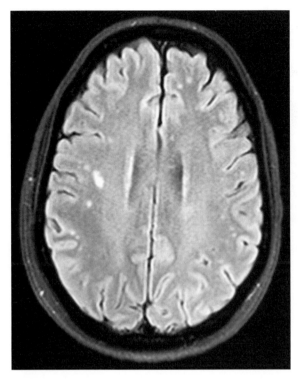

Figure 1.8 Axial MRI brain with multiple areas of non-specific abnormal T2 signal without typical MRI MS lesions.

potentials were normal. Brainstem auditory evoked potentials showed all the waveforms were present on the right side. All the waveforms were absent on the left, which is consistent with severely impaired conduction in the left peripheral auditory pathways.

Three-step assessment

1 Classical clinical features of MS: none; hearing loss is uncommon in MS
2 Neurological examination: consistent with alternative neurological disease; sensorineural hearing loss likely autoimmune
3 Investigations: MRI brain – non-specific changes; MRI cervical and thoracic spine negative; CSF normal; somatosensory and visual evoked potentials negative; peripheral etiology suggested by brainstem auditory evoked potential

   Diagnosis: Suspect isolated autoimmune sensorineural deafness. No convincing evidence of multiple sclerosis.

   Tip: Sudden hearing loss is not a classical clinical symptom of multiple sclerosis and therefore other diagnoses should be actively sought out as

the cause. Oligoclonal bands found on CSF evaluation must be compared with those found on the serum as well. Oligoclonal bands that are unique to the CSF and not present on the serum are considered to be intrathecally produced rather than diffused over from serum and only those oligoclonal bands unique to the CSF are considered to be of diagnostic significance. Brainstem auditory evoked potentials typically are not helpful in the routine assessment of multiple sclerosis. In this case, however, this evaluation showed a clear peripheral nerve defect consistent with autoimmune sensorineural deafness separate from any diagnosis of suspected multiple sclerosis.

Case 6: An elderly patient presenting with gait impairment for possible Parkinson's disease

Although the typical age range for multiple sclerosis is in the teens through the fifth decade, age, in and of itself, should not be the sole determining factor in gauging the possibility that a patient has multiple sclerosis.

A 78-year-old gentleman presented with six years of progressive gait impairment due to lower extremity weakness that was thought to be due to Parkinson's disease. He started to use a walker about five years previously and required a wheelchair about one year ago. While he remained independent in his transfers, he continued to have falls. He had consistent symptoms of neurogenic bladder dysfunction but had no prior history of any acute or subacute neurological episodes with resolution in the past. There was no family history of multiple sclerosis.

On neurological examination, moderate, asymmetric motor weakness was found more on the left than right, both distally in the upper extremities and proximally in the lower extremities. Reflexes were reduced in the lower extremities, but plantar responses were extensor bilaterally. Sensory examination showed marked vibratory sense loss in the lower extremities that was preserved in the hands. He had bilateral circumductive gait consistent with upper motor neuron impairment due to spinal cord disease and could only ambulate with the assistance of a walker.

Brain, cervical and thoracic spinal cord MRIs all demonstrated chronic, non-enhancing T2 weighted

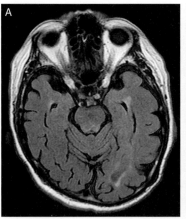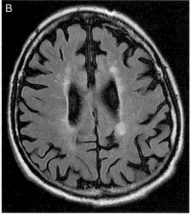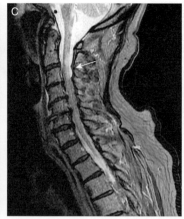

Figure 1.9 A) Axial MRI brain with MS lesions in the temporal horns of the lateral ventricles and periventricular white matter. B) Sagittal T2 MRI cervical spine intramedullary lesions consistent with demyelinating disease most significantly distributed at the C1–C3 levels with central spinal canal stenosis greatest at C5–6 levels.

signal abnormalities highly consistent with multiple sclerosis as the cause for this (Figure 1.9).

Three-step assessment

1 Classical clinical features of MS: progressive myelopathy
2 Neurological examination: consistent with MS
3 Investigations: MRI consistent with MS; CSF not done; EP not done

    Diagnosis: Primary progressive multiple sclerosis with late age of onset.

    Tip: It should be recognized that multiple sclerosis may be diagnosed at an elderly age. Age in and of itself should not be used as a diagnostic indicator for multiple sclerosis. It is suspected that this was the pitfall that led to MS not being considered a diagnostic possibility in this case. The neurological examination with clear evidence of corticospinal tract impairment and sensory loss ruled out Parkinson's disease as a cause in this presented case. A degenerative basal ganglia disease such as Parkinson's disease would not have sensory loss or loss of motor power (despite bradykinesia – slowness of movements) as this case demonstrates.

Further reading

Keegan BM. Therapeutic decision making in a new drug era in multiple sclerosis. *Semin Neurol* 2013;**33**:5–12.

Miller DH, Weinshenker BG, Filippi M, et al. Differential diagnosis of suspected multiple sclerosis: a consensus approach. *MS* 2008;**14**:1157–74.

Polman CH, Reingold SC, Banwell B, et al. Diagnostic criteria for multiple sclerosis: 2010 revisions to the McDonald criteria. *Ann Neurol* 2011;**69**:292–302.

Solomon AJ, Klein EP, Bourdette D. "Undiagnosing" multiple sclerosis: the challenge of misdiagnosis in MS. *Neurology* 2012;**78**:1986–91.

Solomon AJ, Weinshenker BG. Misdiagnosis of multiple sclerosis: frequency, causes, effects, and prevention. *Curr Neurol Neurosci Rep* 2013;**13**:403–10.

Chapter 2

Pitfalls in correctly assessing the clinical course of MS

Introduction

As discussed in Chapter 1, the most critical element in evaluation is making a clear and unequivocal diagnosis of MS using the three-step method: 1) identification of classical clinical features of MS; 2) a neurological examination being either normal or consistent with MS without examining evidence of an alternative neurological disease; and 3) carrying out MRI brain, cervical and thoracic spinal cord investigations, a CSF examination, in particular elevations in oligoclonal bands or the IgG index, and occasionally evoked potentials, serological and other investigations to rule out MS mimickers.

Once you've used the three-step method to identify a definitive diagnosis of multiple sclerosis, the clinician needs to identify the clinical course of multiple sclerosis to assist guiding therapy. Revisions have recently been made to the formal nomenclature of the MS clinical course. At its most broad, the MS clinical course could be dichotomized to relapsing, typically inflammatory MS phenotypes versus progressive, possibly neurodegenerative MS phenotypes. Typical inflammatory clinical courses of MS range from asymptomatic radiologically isolated syndrome (RIS) to inflammatory relapsing forms of multiple sclerosis, including clinically isolated syndrome (CIS) and relapsing-remitting multiple sclerosis (RRMS) (Table 2.1). These patients do not have progressive impairment in between attacks and any impairment is solely due to acute relapses and prior relapses with incomplete recovery. In contrast, patients with primary progressive multiple sclerosis (PPMS) and secondary progressive multiple sclerosis (SPMS) show progressive neurological deterioration in between attacks that do not appear to be due to typical inflammatory disease. Importantly, immunomodulatory medications currently available for multiple sclerosis do not appear to have a robust treatment effect on progressive forms of multiple sclerosis and treat typical inflammation that causes clinical attacks and new MRI lesions of the relapsing forms of multiple sclerosis.

RIS is diagnosed in patients without characteristic clinical cardinal symptoms or signs of MS attacks or of progressive MS who are found to have MRI lesions highly typical of MS. MRI examinations have usually been performed for reasons such as a headache, unrelated trauma, and healthy controls for MRI research protocols. Further investigations, such as a CSF examination, may reveal asymptomatic spinal cord lesions and abnormalities consistent with MS (elevated unique CSF oligoclonal bands and/or IgG index). While patients with RIS are at risk for a future clinical CNS demyelinating attack or progressive CNS disease diagnostic of MS (~30 percent over 5 years), currently treatment is not recommended in most RIS cases. CIS is diagnosed in patients with a single clinical demyelinating attack without further MRI findings of dissemination in time of simultaneous new and "active" (T1 gadolinium-enhancing) and older and "inactive" (T2 lesions without gadolinium enhancement) MS lesions. RRMS is diagnosed in patients who have either two or more clinical demyelinating attacks or a single clinical attack accompanied by MRI evidence of inflammatory disease activity, disseminated in time and space within the CNS (i.e. new and "active" (T1 gadolinium-enhancing) and older and "inactive" (T2 lesions without gadolinium enhancement) MS lesions) that distinguish it from CIS. RRMS patients must have no clinical evidence of clinical worsening between MS attacks that cannot be attributed to acute inflammatory disease (i.e. acute relapses and incomplete recovery from prior relapses). SPMS is diagnosed in patients who have had at least one definite acute clinical MS attack in the past (with or without full recovery), with insidiously progressive neurological impairment (typically myelopathic gait disorder) not entirely due to new inflammatory activity (i.e. new MS attacks or marked new MRI

Table 2.1 Clinical courses typical of multiple sclerosis

Clinical Course	Classical clinical MS relapse(s)	Progressive MS impairment not due to MS relapses	Comment
Radiologically isolated syndrome (RIS)	0	No	MRI findings highly typical of MS without classical clinical features of MS relapses or progression
Clinically isolated syndrome (CIS)	1	No	One clinical relapse without concomitant gadolinium-enhancing and non-enhancing MS lesions on MRI fulfilling dissemination in time and location in CNS
Relapsing-remitting multiple sclerosis (RRMS)	≥1	No	May have more than one relapse or one relapse with other asymptomatic concomitant gadolinium-enhancing and non-enhancing MS MRI lesions fulfilling dissemination in time and location in CNS
Secondary progressive multiple sclerosis (SPMS)	≥1	Yes	Progressive MS impairment not due to MS relapses with at least one and typically many prior clinical relapses with improvement (each relapse improvement may be incomplete)
Primary progressive multiple sclerosis (PPMS)	0	Yes	Progressive MS impairment not due to MS relapses without any prior clinical relapse

lesions). PPMS patients present with progressive myelopathic gait dysfunction, cerebellar ataxia or cognitive impairment due to MS without any history of ever having even a single acute clinical attack in the past. To fulfill diagnostic criteria for PPMS, the progression must be of one year's duration and have brain and spinal cord MRI abnormalities and/or CSF examination consistent with MS. Given the lack of a major contributor of typical inflammatory activity in SPMS and PPMS, current MS immunomodulatory medications are mostly ineffective.

Case 7: A woman with headaches and typical brain demyelinating lesions on MRI. Is it relapsing-remitting MS or radiologically isolated syndrome?

A 44-year-old woman presented with migraine headaches and was found to have brain MRI abnormalities. She had never experienced typical classical features of acute clinical attacks of multiple sclerosis. Specifically, she had never had symptoms of optic neuritis, significant binocular diplopia, dysarthria, dysphagia, hemiparesis, hemisensory deficit, Lhermitte symptoms or progressive myelopathic gait impairment. On one occasion, she had a brief episode of numbness in the left lower leg lasting only one hour, which resolved spontaneously and never reoccurred.

A brain MRI was carried out entirely due to a history of migraine headaches and showed areas of abnormal signal consistent with CNS demyelinating disease (Figure 2.1). A CSF examination was performed on two separate occasions, with no oligoclonal bands found on either of the evaluations. Minimal IgG index elevations of 0.75 and another at 0.76 were found where the local lab high diagnostic cutoff value was 0.6 (note: many lab IgG normal values are ≤ 0.85).

Repeat brain MRIs continued to show areas of abnormal signal but no interval development of any new lesions. There were juxtacortical lesions, a subcortical lesion in the left hemisphere white

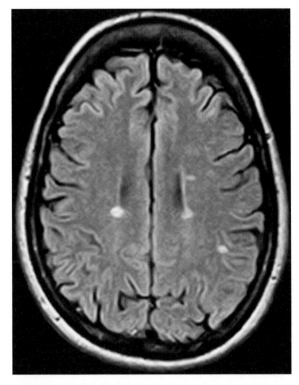

Figure 2.1 Axial FLAIR MRI brain showing ovoid, periventricular and juxtacortical lesions also involving the corpus callosum highly characteristic of MS lesions in this patient without classical clinical features of MS.

matter and a posterior left frontal lobe lesion. Cervical and thoracic spine MRI scans were normal with no evidence of demyelination within the spinal cord. Somatosensory evoked potentials were normal. EMG and nerve conduction studies were normal.

Three-step assessment

1 Classical clinical features of MS: none
2 Neurological examination: normal
3 Investigations: MRI brain consistent with MS; MRI spinal cord normal; CSF abnormalities (elevated IgG index) consistent with MS

Diagnosis: Radiologically isolated syndrome (RIS).

Tip: A detailed clinical history should check for classical cardinal clinical features for suspected relapses of multiple sclerosis or of a progressive neurological deficit consistent with progressive multiple sclerosis. The absence of these clinical features, along with highly characteristic brain

and/or spinal cord MRI lesions, is consistent with a diagnosis of RIS.

The radiologically isolated syndrome is a relatively recent concept. Research groups studying this have shown that the risk of developing one clinical attack consistent with multiple sclerosis is approximately 30–35 percent within the first five years of evaluation. As was the case in the presented history, MRI scans are generally recommended for such procedures as migraine headache evaluation, routine follow-up for executive clinical evaluation, being a control in an investigational MRI study, and investigation of other nonspecific symptoms. Patients with asymptomatic typical demyelinating lesions within the spinal cord are at a higher risk for a future clinical attack than those without spinal cord MRI lesions. Currently, immunomodulatory MS medications are not generally recommended for this patient group.

Case 8: A patient with fatigue and a history of remote neurological symptoms, but without significant neurological debility. Could this be benign MS?

Some patients appear to have rather "benign" forms of multiple sclerosis. Definitions of this MS clinical course differ; however, it is often loosely defined as a lack of significant neurological impairment at least 15 to 20 years following the onset of multiple sclerosis. This should be distinguished from radiologically isolated syndrome, where there are *no* classical symptoms of clinical MS attacks but highly typical MRI features are found incidentally. In benign multiple sclerosis, patients definitively have multiple sclerosis with at least one prior attack and new MRI lesions occurring but seem to accrue little or no impairment with or without immunomodulatory medications, even after decades of having the disease. Benign multiple sclerosis remains controversial as MS-related cognitive impairment may be underreported, and long-term follow-up in some patients is limited to fully assess this.

A 67-year-old gentleman presented because of troublesome fatigue. He came with an existing "possible" diagnosis of multiple sclerosis. In the 1970s, the patient experienced an episode of painless, binocular diplopia lasting three months with resolution. In 1980, the patient developed a Lhermitte symptom accompanied by a sense of leg heaviness. Since then, he described waxing and waning sensory symptoms including tongue burning and numb spots on the face, left lower abdomen and left foot. There were other widely distributed patches of sensory symptoms that were rare and difficult to describe. There was no recent history to suggest any classical clinical relapses of multiple sclerosis. He was very active and was able to run without difficulty and walk for miles without any gait impairment.

On neurological examination his mental status was found to be normal, as were his visual fields. Extraocular movements were also entirely normal, with no internuclear ophthalmoplegia. A motor exam was entirely normal and plantar responses were flexor bilaterally.

A brain MRI showed multiple areas of abnormal signal highly consistent with MS, and was unchanged from a brain MRI performed fifteen years previously (Figure 2.2). There was little or no change in the number, size or signal intensity of the lesions seen. A spinal cord MRI showed a small focus of abnormal

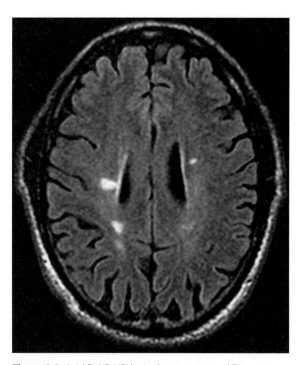

Figure 2.2 Axial FLAIR MRI brain showing scattered T2 hyperintensities, predominantly within the periventricular white matter compatible with clinical diagnosis of multiple sclerosis.

T2 signal intensity at the C2–C3 level consistent with multiple sclerosis (not shown).

Three-step assessment

1 Classical clinical features of MS: brainstem attack with diplopia, Lhermitte symptom with cervical myelopathy
2 Neurological examination: normal
3 Investigations: MRI brain and cervical spine consistent with MS; CSF not performed

Diagnosis: Benign relapsing-remitting multiple sclerosis.

Tip: Despite experiencing few problems over many decades, the patient clearly has relapsing-remitting multiple sclerosis, which is confirmed by his clinical history as well as MRI investigations. MRI scans compared with many years before may show little or no ongoing or intervening inflammatory activity in those with benign MS. Patients may go many years or decades without clear significant neurological impairment or confirmed secondary progressive multiple sclerosis.

Case 9: MS with occasional symptomatic worsening. Is it relapsing-remitting or a progressive clinical course of MS?

Pseudo exacerbations are temporarily worsened old MS symptoms that occur in association with increased body temperature, fatigue, infection or stress. This is a heralding of old symptoms due to inactive demyelinated multiple sclerosis plaques rather than an acute inflammatory attack of multiple sclerosis. Pseudo exacerbations of multiple sclerosis may occur with most MS clinical courses but are particularly common in patients with progressive forms of multiple sclerosis of long disease duration who have established disability. Occasionally the symptoms may be significant and prolonged. Treatment aimed at curing infection or reducing body temperature and returning to baseline neurological status is important but this does not constitute new inflammatory relapses of MS.

A 57-year-old woman had initial symptoms of multiple sclerosis with loss of sensation in her lower extremities for three weeks with spontaneous resolution at age 30 following the birth of one of her children. A brain MRI scan and CSF examination were convincing for the diagnosis of multiple sclerosis. One sister had MS and used a walker.

She did not recall symptoms of prior optic neuritis nor of diplopia, and could not recall other definite attacks over time since the post-partum period. She had symptoms and signs of neurogenic bowel and bladder dysfunction. She described a steady decline in her gait due to progressive motor weakness over a number of years. She started to use a walker five years ago. She did not use a cane before that, but she did have significant imbalance. She now uses a scooter and a wheelchair at home. She had initiated treatment with interferon beta-1b, which she has remained on for ten years. She has had therapeutic intolerance with significant injection site reactions, and expressed a desired to discontinue immunomodulatory MS medications.

On examination, her mental status was normal. Her cranial nerves were normal, and her speech was clear. On motor examination, she had weakness on the right greater than left upper and lower extremities in an upper motor neuron "pyramidal" distribution. Reflexes were brisker on the right than left, and her plantar responses were extensor bilaterally. Vibratory sense was impaired in the lower extremities. She walked with a markedly impaired spastic ataxic gait, right more than left, and required a walker for standing.

A brain MRI remained entirely stable with areas of abnormal signal consistent with multiple sclerosis, as serial brain MRIs from the past had shown (Figure 2.3). A cervical spinal cord MRI showed areas of abnormal T2 signal without gadolinium-enhancing lesions, which is consistent with chronic demyelination of multiple sclerosis.

Three-step assessment

1 Classical clinical features of MS: progressive myelopathy following resolved acute sensory myelopathy
2 Neurological examination: consistent with MS: quadriparesis with corticospinal tract impairment and sensory loss
3 Investigations: brain MRI consistent with MS, positive without new changes over time; cervical spine MRI consistent with MS without new changes over time; CSF consistent with MS

Diagnosis: Secondary progressive multiple sclerosis.

Tip: Patients presenting with a history of at least one prior demyelinating attack, a very long history of

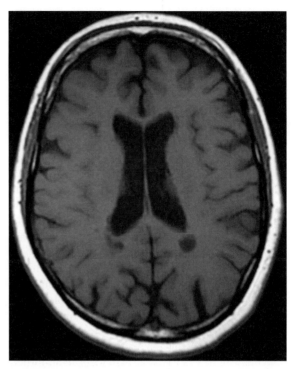

Figure 2.3 Axial T1 MRI brain showing chronic, inactive, ovoid areas of T1 hypointensity ("black holes") consistent with chronic MS; multiple focal and confluent areas of hyperintense T2 signal change were also seen, as well as hyperintense T2 signal change within the pons (not shown).

multiple sclerosis with progressive gait disorder, entirely stable neuroimaging over time and no recent symptoms of definite attacks is diagnostic of secondary progressive multiple sclerosis. Patients with secondary progressive MS, however, may have pseudo-exacerbations usually associated with infection, high body temperature or fatigue that can cause definite and occasionally profound symptomatic worsening. This is presumably due to relatively noninflammatory, pre-existing, demyelination from longstanding MS. Relapsing-remitting multiple sclerosis is responsive to immunomodulatory medications, whereas secondary progressive multiple sclerosis without recent clinical relapses or ongoing inflammation in MRI scans are not robustly responsive to these existing therapies.

Case 10: A patient with a history of resolved gait impairment. Is it secondary progressive MS?

A 59-year-old woman was evaluated for possible secondary progressive multiple sclerosis. She was diagnosed with multiple sclerosis ten years previously when she had symptoms of low back pain, and numbness and paresthesias of the arms and left leg. She had word-finding difficulties without any symptoms suggesting more significant memory loss. She had never had other symptoms suggestive of optic neuritis or significant diplopia. There was no family history of multiple sclerosis or other neurological disease. She did report gait imbalance in the past and used a cane for two years prior to evaluation. She then used two walking sticks and had an ankle-foot orthosis on one side. She then started walking more frequently to increase her exercise endurance and now had returned successfully to walking about five miles; she was limited here only by shortness of breath but not by motor weakness, and she used no gait aids.

A prior brain MRI performed locally was interpreted there to show T2 signal abnormalities thought to be suggestive changes of multiple sclerosis. Cervical spine MRIs performed on different occasions was alternately interpreted to either show evidence of multiple sclerosis or to be normal,

with only artifactual changes seen. A CSF examination had not been performed, nor had evoked potentials.

The patient initiated glatiramer acetate and was on it for ten years. She was then changed to natalizumab, which she took for six months but then discontinued it when the JC virus serological antibody tested positive; other immunomodulatory medications were discontinued at that time. While it was considered that she likely had a secondary progressive MS course, fingolimod was recommended despite it not being approved for secondary progressive MS.

A brain MRI performed on her evaluation did not show any highly suggestive evidence of MS (Figure 2.4). A cervical spine MRI was normal. A CSF examination was performed and was normal without elevations in the IgG index or oligoclonal bands.

Three-step assessment

1 Classical clinical features of MS: none, suspected progressive gait impairment; sustained,

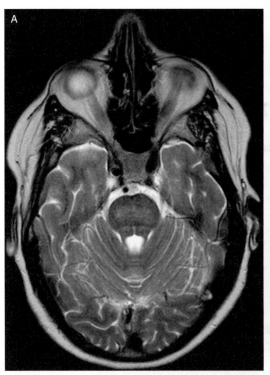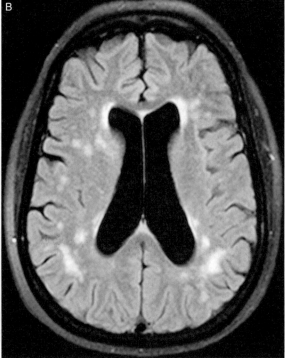

Figure 2.4 Axial T2 and FLAIR MRI brain with moderate areas of nonspecific signal abnormality in the pons and brain most suggestive of small vessel ischemic disease. No typical MS lesions were found in the corpus callosum or middle cerebellar peduncles (not shown).

marked improvement was inconsistent with progressive MS

2 Neurological examination: normal

3 Investigations: brain MRI – non-specific changes; spinal cord MRI normal; CSF normal

Diagnosis: Not multiple sclerosis and nothing to suggest secondary progressive multiple sclerosis.

Tip: Secondary progressive multiple sclerosis is evaluated on a clinical basis, both from the clinical history the patient provides and, where possible, by repeatedly performing neurological examinations over time. True secondary progressive MS, when established and long term, is not considered reversible and the sustained marked improvement described in this case would not be compatible with this. The diagnosis of multiple sclerosis must be reevaluated critically in such cases. As non-specific brain MRI lesions are so common, high-quality radiological interpretations, a high-quality spinal cord MRI and evaluation of CSF and occasionally evoked potentials are critical to secure a diagnosis of MS.

Case 11: A woman with vertigo, diplopia and head pain. Is it relapsing-remitting MS?

A 34-year-old woman was evaluated for complaints of head pain and an abnormal brain MRI scan.

Four months prior to presentation, she developed true spinning vertigo with simultaneous horizontal, binocular, painless diplopia lasting 48 hours continuously followed by spontaneous resolution. She subsequently developed a severe posterior headache that required narcotic analgesics. She had no history suggestive of other clinical attacks of multiple sclerosis or gait impairment. She had a history of jaw pain diagnosed as osteoarthritis. There was no family history of multiple sclerosis.

Her neurological examination was entirely normal.

A brain MRI showed multiple areas of non-enhancing abnormal T2 signal consistent with multiple sclerosis (Figure 2.5). A cervical spine MRI was normal, while a thoracic spine MRI was not performed. A CSF examination showed four unique CSF oligoclonal bands.

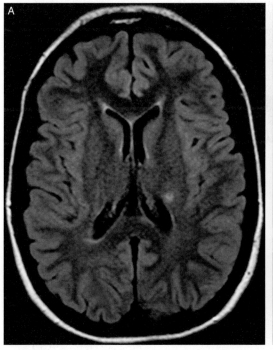
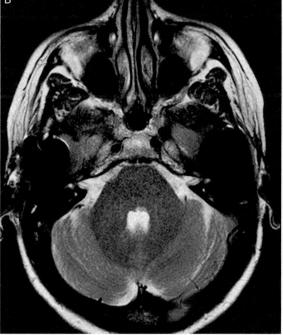

Figure 2.5 Brain MRI.

Three-step assessment

1 Classical clinical features of MS: brainstem attack with vertigo and binocular, painless diplopia
2 Neurological examination: normal
3 Investigations: Brain MRI consistent with MS; CSF consistent with CNS demyelinating disease

Diagnosis: Clinically isolated syndrome with high risk MRI findings for future development of multiple sclerosis.

Tip: The patient's history of painless binocular diplopia lasting 48 hours was consistent with a demyelinating attack, and the brain MRI findings were highly compelling. Given that there were more than two additional areas of abnormal signal consistent with CNS demyelination, it put her at a high risk of developing definitive relapsing-remitting multiple sclerosis with subsequent attacks. She would qualify for injectable immunomodulatory medications aimed at multiple sclerosis at this time. Occasionally, some patients take a watchful waiting approach and repeat neuroimaging in 6 to 12 months could be performed if they remained clinically asymptomatic. If there are no clinical symptoms of attacks of multiple sclerosis, repeat neuroimaging and reconsideration of immunomodulatory medications should be carried out. It is important to go over the clinical features of attacks of multiple sclerosis with patients so that they know what would be important to identify.

Pain is of uncertain relevance to CNS demyelinating disease in this patient. The symptoms of head pain and possible occipital neuralgia would not necessarily be associated with new demyelination, although the brainstem spinal trigeminal tracts can be involved leading to this type of pain in rare patients.

Further reading

Clinical Course of MS

Lublin FD, Reingold SC. Defining the clinical course of multiple sclerosis: Results of an international survey. *Neurology* 1996;**46**:907–11.

FD L, SC R, JA C, et al. Defining the clinical course of multiple sclerosis: the 2013 revisions. *Neurology* 2014;**83**: 278–86.

RIS

Okuda DT, Siva A, Kantarci O, et al. Radiologically isolated syndrome: 5-year risk for an initial clinical event. *PLoS One* 2014;**9**:e90509.

Okuda DT, Mowry EM, Cree BAC, et al. Asymptomatic spinal cord lesions predict disease progression in radiologically isolated syndrome. *Neurology* 2011;**76**: 686–92.

CIS

Miller D, Barkhof F, Montalban X, Thompson A, Filippi M. Clinically isolated syndromes suggestive of multiple sclerosis, part I: natural history, pathogenesis, diagnosis, and prognosis. *Lancet Neurol* 2005;**4**:281–8.

Miller D, Barkhof F, Montalban X, Thompson A, Filippi M. Clinically isolated syndromes suggestive of multiple sclerosis, part 2: non-conventional MRI, recovery processes, and management. *Lancet Neurol* 2005;**4**:341–8.

Montalban X, Tintore M, Swanton J, et al. MRI criteria for MS in patients with clinically isolated syndromes. *Neurology* 2010;**74**:427–34.

PPMS

Miller DH, Leary SM. Primary-progressive multiple sclerosis. *Lancet Neurol* 2007;**6**:903–12.

Pitfalls in recognizing uncommon MS clinical presentations

Introduction

Prior chapters have described highly characteristic and classical features of multiple sclerosis relapses and progressive neurological impairment that are helpful in diagnosing MS and identifying its clinical course in the vast majority of cases. Some MS symptoms, while remaining very characteristic, are far less frequent but should still alert the clinician to a diagnosis of multiple sclerosis, and these will be described here.

MS may cause paroxysmal symptoms that are distinctive. While acute inflammatory relapses of multiple sclerosis generally last at least 24 hours in duration and more commonly last days to weeks, paroxysmal symptoms may last only seconds to minutes. Paroxysmal symptoms of MS are usually stereotyped and repetitive, and therefore may be mistaken for an epileptiform etiology. It is felt that many paroxysmal MS symptoms are due to ephaptic transmission (cross-talk) between demyelinated neurons.

Case 12: Repetitive painful spasms of the left arm and leg. Is it multiple sclerosis?

A 49-year-old woman was originally evaluated eight years earlier when she had left upper and lower extremity weakness, with dysarthria and gait incoordination. On her initial evaluations, both MRI and CSF investigations were consistent with multiple sclerosis as the cause. She received intravenous corticosteroids for MS attacks on three subsequent occasions, each time resulting in an improvement back to normal, and took chronic immunomodulatory MS treatment with glatiramer acetate.

On this occasion she presented because she had developed left upper and lower extremity painful flexor spasms that repetitively occurred up to 45 times per day. An unusual sensation in the arm would precede them, but despite that she could not voluntarily abort the spasm. She initiated carbamazepine by mouth, resulting in initial, but incomplete, improvement.

On neurological examination she had minimal gait ataxia with and mild bilateral vibratory sense loss in the toes. Repetitive, involuntary left upper and lower extremity spasms were observed.

A brain MRI showed multiple abnormal areas of abnormal signal consistent with MS. A single focus in the posterior limb of the right internal capsule demonstrated gadolinium enhancement and restricted diffusion consistent with an acute demyelinating MS plaque (Figure 3.1).

Three-step assessment

1 Classical clinical features of MS: painful tonic spasms prior to brainstem attacks
2 Neurological examination: consistent with MS: a gait ataxia with distal vibratory sense loss; paroxysmal spasms observed
3 Investigations: MRI brain consistent with MS with acute demyelinating plaque, CSF consistent with MS

Tip: Paroxysmal painful tonic spasms may be due to CNS demyelination. The stereotyped and repetitive nature of the spells, as well as the frequency (which in this case amounted to up to 45 times per day), is characteristic of this condition, and this frequency may rule out an epileptiform cause as well. Usually the inciting demyelinating lesion is found within the cervical spine, but lesions in the internal capsule, as was the case in this patient, may also cause this symptom. Antiepileptic drugs improve MS paroxysmal spasms and exquisite therapeutic responsiveness to carbamazepine is common. An increased dose of carbamazepine was required in this patient, who subsequently experienced complete elimination of the paroxysmal tonic spasms. Often carbamazepine can be weaned and discontinued successfully after weeks to months of therapy, with the spasms having abated for a prolonged duration.

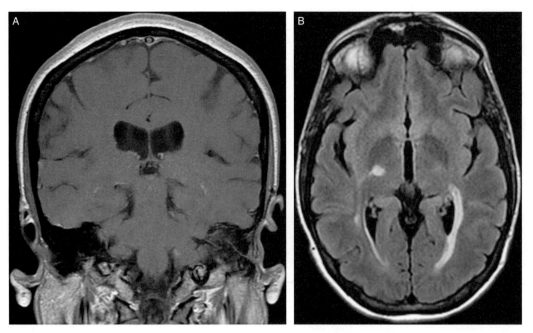

Figure 3.1 Axial FLAIR, coronal T1 with gadolinium MRI brain multiple demyelinating plaques consistent with multiple sclerosis within the white matter of both cerebral hemispheres, with single enhancing focus posterior limb right internal capsule consistent with an acute demyelinating plaque.

Case 13: A man with treatment-resistant trigeminal neuralgia

A 64-year-old gentleman was evaluated who had been symptomatic from first and third division right trigeminal neuralgia for six years. Over that period, the painful symptoms had waxed and waned in severity. Triggers such as eating provoked the symptoms and he described the pain as like "lightning," with a severity estimated at 8/10 on a Likert pain scale. He had been treated with gabapentin and carbamazepine for years on increasing doses as he experienced more frequent, and more severe, lancinating pain episodes. It was considered to be routine trigeminal neuralgia and he came with no prior brain MRI or other neurological diagnosis at the time.

He had no cognitive symptoms or memory loss. He had mild diplopia due to remote trauma at 18 years of age. He had no dysphagia, dysarthria or other cranial nerve symptoms. He had no symptoms of motor weakness, gait difficulties or incoordination or sensory loss.

On neurological examination he had normal cranial nerve examination with mild distal left upper extremity weakness with left hyperreflexia and left extensor plantar response.

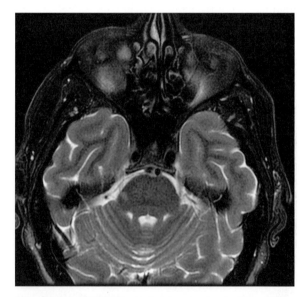

Figure 3.2 Axial T2 MRI brain showing prominent white matter lesion within the right aspect of the pons at the root entry zone of the right trigeminal nerve. A number of ovoid T2 hyperintense and T1 hypointense white matter lesions and T2 hyperintense lesions were seen within the cervical spinal cord (not shown).

A brain MRI showed T2 hyperintense foci within the cerebral hemispheric white matter with a discrete focus of T2 hyperintensity within the right pons at the trigeminal nerve root entry zone (Figure 3.2).

A cervical spinal cord MRI showed non-nenhancing, short-segment T2 hyperintense intramedullary lesions, all of which are consistent with MS.

Three-step assessment

1 Classical clinical features of MS: trigeminal neuralgia
2 Neurological examination consistent with MS: left corticospinal tract impairment (upper motor neuron weakness with extensor plantar response)
3 Investigations: MRI brain consistent with MS with lesion at trigeminal nerve root entry zone; MRI cervical spine consistent with MS

Tip: Trigeminal neuralgia may be the heralding symptom of MS as it was in this presented case. A brain MRI is recommended in all patients with trigeminal neuralgia to identify any vascular compression that causes "typical" primary trigeminal neuralgia, as well as to investigate the possibility of a secondary etiology such as MS as a cause. Trigeminal neuralgia may be bilateral in some MS patients. Surgical management of MS-related TN relies more on ablative therapies rather than vascular decompressive surgery given the etiology of demyelination at the trigeminal nerve root entry zone as opposed to being from arterial compression of the nerve.

Case 14:   A man with recurrent spells of ataxia and dysarthria

A 39-year-old man presented with recurrent symptoms of imbalance. Many years ago he had numbness involving the left axilla, trunk and left leg that resolved spontaneously after four days, consistent with an inflammatory sensory cervical myelopathy. He had no prior episodes of ataxia, optic neuritis, diplopia, dysphagia or unilateral motor symptoms. He then developed repetitive and stereotypical spells. For approximately five to ten seconds, he would have an aura that "something is happening." Following that he would have 30-second spells where his speech would be very "effortful" and slurred, without mental confusion or aphasia. Toward the end of each spell, he would experience left leg and arm tingling paresthesias. The symptoms would always proceed exactly in this stereotyped fashion and occurred repetitively a few times every hour.

He had never awoken from sleep due to these spells and there were no identifiable provoking factors.

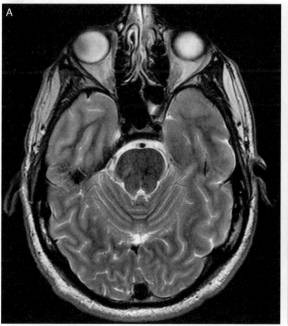
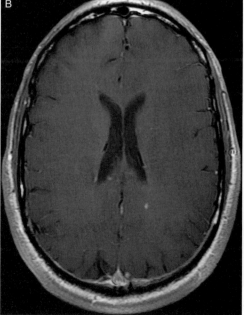

Figure 3.3 A) Axial T2 MRI brain showing linear signal abnormality in the right pons; patchy T2 signal hyperintensity was also noted within the brainstem around the obex and along the left lateral cervical medullary junction. B) Axial T1 with gadolinium MRI brain with enhancing lesion in right hemispheric white matter.

His neurological examination was normal.

A brain MRI demonstrated multiple white matter T2 hyperintensities, several of which were gadolinium enhancing (Figure 3.3). A cervical spine MRI demonstrated multiple non-enhancing lesions consistent with MS. Thoracic spine MRI and CSF examinations were not performed. EEGs during two typical spells showed no epileptiform activity.

Three-step assessment

1 Classical clinical features of MS: sensory myelopathy with resolution, paroxysmal ataxia and dysarthria
2 Neurological examination: normal
3 Investigations: MRI brain consistent with MS; MRI cervical spine consistent with MS

Tip: Paroxysmal symptoms of ataxia and dysarthria are an uncommon manifestation of MS. The suspected cause is due to ephaptic transmission (cross talk) over demyelinated axons similar to painful tonic spasms of MS and MS-related trigeminal neuralgia. Typically the location of the MS lesion responsible for this presentation is within the brainstem or cerebellar white matter pathways.

Case 15: Recurrent encephalopathy in a patient with longstanding MS

A 79-year-old woman had a history of MS for over 40 years. Initially she had an attack-related disease, with acute and initially resolving symptoms mostly referable to within the spinal cord. She started to use a cane 38 years ago and had been wheelchair bound for the last 30 years. Over the last 25 years she was unable to transfer independently.

She was evaluated repeatedly in the emergency room for recurrent symptoms of confusion and drowsiness consistent with significant encephalopathy with some hearing impairment and slurred dysarthric speech. During an outpatient visit by her primary care provider a reliable body temperature could not be recorded. She was sent to the emergency room, where an initial body temperature was recorded at 32.1 degrees Celsius. She was rewarmed with IV fluids, and it improved to 35.2 degrees Celsius.

On neurological examination, she had a right internuclear ophthalmoplegia, upper motor neuron quadriparesis and was wheelchair bound.

Prior brain and spinal cord MRIs showed typical changes of chronic demyelination due to MS (Figure 3.4). A prior CSF examination showed eight

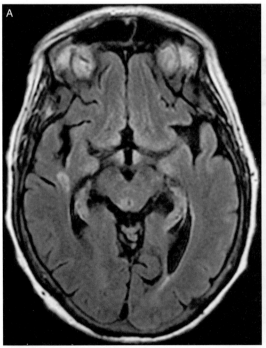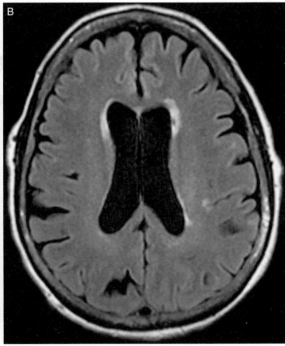

Figure 3.4 Axial FLAIR MRI brain showing periventricular signal abnormality consistent with MS. Abnormal multifocal patchy cervical and thoracic cord T2 hyperintensities with focal thoracic cord atrophy consistent with demyelinating disease were also seen (not shown).

unique CSF oligoclonal bands. A CT angiogram showed no significant abnormalities. An EEG showed atypical triphasic waves and mild slowing posteriorly with no potentially epileptogenic activity consistent with a non-specific encephalopathy.

Three-step assessment

1 Classical clinical features of MS: MS–associated hypothermia causing recurrent encephalopathy; myelopathy with severe progressive impairment
2 Neurological examination: consistent with MS: upper motor neuron quadriparesis with internuclear ophthalmoplegia (INO)
3 Investigations: MRI brain consistent with MS; MRI spine consistent with MS; CSF consistent with MS

Tip: MS-associated hypothermia causing recurrent encephalopathy is an uncommon presentation. Brain MRIs occasionally may show hypothalamic involvement but this is not seen in all cases. Particularly with patients with long-term multiple sclerosis with recurring encephalopathy, checking the core body temperature is critical to assess for possible hypothermia. Warming toward normal body temperature improves symptoms. Guarding against recurring drops in body temperature is crucial to avoiding significant encephalopathy recurrence.

Case 16: A man with recurrent right lower extremity weakness fluctuating with neck movement

A 57-year-old gentleman presented with a two-year history of progressive, but markedly fluctuating, right lower extremity weakness. The patient noticed that when he engaged in increased physical activity such as climbing on and off tractors he would get a sense of diffuse weakness as well as more focal weakness of the right lower extremity. His symptoms were more easily provoked during hot summer months and when his job-related exertion would cause him to get overheated, and he noticed a strong association of the symptoms with neck position. Specifically, neck hyperextension instantly caused transient improvement in the right lower extremity weakness. In addition to this, if he flexed his neck while putting on his trousers he would suddenly lose right leg strength and he could not flex his hip to get them on. He did not have a typical sensory Lhermitte symptom on neck flexion.

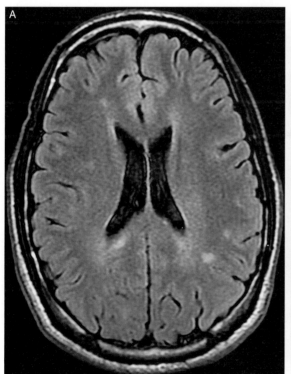
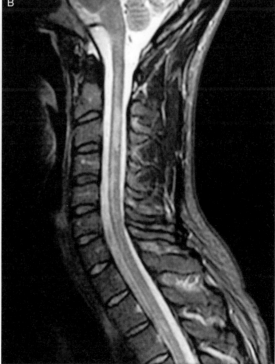

Figure 3.5 A) Axial FLAIR MRI brain with callosal and juxtacortical MS lesions. B) Sagittal T2 MRI cervical spine showing multifocal T2 hyperintense lesions within the cervical spinal cord compatible with multiple sclerosis.

His symptoms gradually progressed as the day wore on with worsened limping and catching of the right toe. He noticed heaviness and clumsiness in the right arm and hand, which again was particularly worse in the hot weather months and better when he worked in cooler weather and got less overheated.

Four years prior to these symptoms he had binocular, painless diplopia that resolved in six weeks and was diagnosed as left lateral rectus muscle weakness without further clarifying etiology being found.

On neurological examination, with the neck in neutral position he had mild strength impairment in the right lower extremity. With neck hyperextension it promptly improved, but did not entirely normalize compared to the left side. With neck hyperflexion there was marked definite worsening of the right lower extremity strength within a couple of seconds. Further, after 10 or 20 seconds of hyperventilation, he also would experience transient improvement in right lower extremity strength.

Brain and spinal cord MRIs showed numerous areas of abnormal T2 signal without gadolinium enhancement consistent with MS (Figure 3.5). CSF examination showed an elevated IgG index and five unique oligoclonal bands. An EMG study was normal.

Three-step assessment

1 Classical clinical features of MS: McArdle's sign with worsening motor impairment on neck flexion, history of binocular, painless diplopia with resolution
2 Neurological examination: myelopathic clinical findings and inducible McArdle's sign consistent with MS
3 Investigations: MRI brain consistent with MS; MRI spine consistent with MS; CSF consistent with MS

Diagnosis: Secondary progressive MS; McArdle's sign due to CNS demyelination in the cervical spine.

Tip: Significant worsening of motor impairment on neck movement may suggest CNS demyelination such as multiple sclerosis as the cause. McArdle's sign is well documented, particularly in patients with long-term multiple sclerosis. It may, however, be a heralding feature of multiple sclerosis.

Case 17: A man with fluctuating, then progressive, visual impairment

A 25-year-old right-handed man presented with right eye symptoms that had been present for several years.

He could not describe specifically the circumstances surrounding their onset or time course. He described it as "haziness" of vision in his right eye as though he is "looking through a film or frosted glass." He underwent optometric evaluation but the visual haziness was not correctable by refractive changes. The visual symptom was stable until one day, while practicing archery, he became aware that he could no longer distinguish the rings of the target with his right eye. He then checked his vision by looking in a mirror and found that with his left eye vision was normal, but with his right eye he could only see his outline without color or contrast. His vision returned to his baseline right visual haziness after approximately two or three hours. For the next few days he had recurrence of the symptoms with subsequent resolution after two or three hours. The patient reported ongoing, but intermittent, worsening of his right visual disturbance. When he awakens in the morning he has only slight haziness of vision in his right eye. If he were to engage in activities during the day that raise his body temperature, such as drinking several cups of hot coffee, exercising, becoming emotionally distressed or being out in bright sunlight, he will notice that his vision again worsens to be "completely whited out."

After two years of follow-up, he noted similar visual problems with exercise, this time involving the left eye decompensating to about 85 percent normal with significant exertion and heat. His right eye would go from about 85 percent at baseline in ambient temperatures down to about 25 percent with significant exertion. He then developed progressive left leg weakness. Previously gait impairment would occur only after a very long period of walking of about 60 minutes but now might impair him after about 15 minutes. He had a five-year history of erectile dysfunction with urinary hesitancy.

On neurological evaluation, visual field examination revealed a central scotoma in the right eye only, with visual acuity of 20/40 in the right eye and 20/20 in the left eye and significant color vision impairment in the right eye only. There was a right-sided relative afferent pupillary defect. Disk color was normal bilaterally, as were extraocular movements. The rest of the exam was normal.

A brain MRI showed typical areas of abnormal T2 signal of MS without any orbital lesions. A spinal cord MRI was not performed. A CSF examination showed an elevated IgG index and elevated oligoclonal bands. An MR angiogram and MR venography were normal.

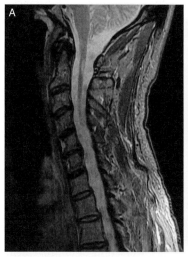 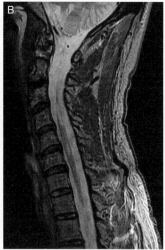 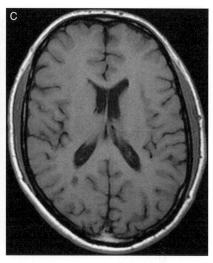

Figure 3.6 A) Sagittal T2 MRI cervical spine showing multifocal T2 hyperintense lesions within the cervical spinal cord compatible with multiple sclerosis. B) Axial T1 MRI brain showing an ovoid chronic, inactive, area of T1 hypointensity ("black hole") consistent with chronic MS.

Three-step assessment

1 Classical clinical features of MS: Uhthoff phenomenon, both eyes sequentially, progressive myelopathy with progressive gait impairment
2 Neurological examination: optic neuropathy consistent with MS
3 Investigations: MRI brain consistent with MS; CSF consistent with MS

   Diagnosis: MS with Uhthoff phenomenon

   Tip: Uhthoff phenomenon is transient dimming or obscuring of vision associated with an elevated body temperature. This may be induced by exercise, fatigue, infection, fever or other forms of heat exposure. This symptom may be improved with rest and cooling of the core body temperature and does not generally indicate a new inflammatory demyelinating attack. Symptom resolution usually occurs within 15–20 minutes of cooling.

Further reading

O'Neill JH, Mills KR, Murray NM. McArdle's sign in multiple sclerosis. Journal of Neurology. *Neurosurgery & Psychiatry*; **50**:1691–3.

Frohman TC, Davis SL, Beh S, Greenberg BM, Remington G, Frohman EM. Uhthoff's phenomena in MS–clinical features and pathophysiology. *Nat Rev Neurol* 2013;**9**:535–40.

Park K, Tanaka K, Tanaka M. Uhthoff's phenomenon in multiple sclerosis and neuromyelitis optica. *Eur Neurol* 2014;**72**:153–6.

Smith KJ, McDonald WI. The pathophysiology of multiple sclerosis: the mechanisms underlying the production of symptoms and the natural history of the disease. *Philos Trans R Soc Lond B Biol Sci* 1999;**354**:1649–73.

van Diemen HA, van Dongen MM, Dammers JW, Polman CH. Increased visual impairment after exercise (Uhthoff's phenomenon) in multiple sclerosis: therapeutic possibilities. *Eur Neurol* 1992;**32**:231–4.

Iorio R, Capone F, Plantone D, Batocchi AP. Paroxysmal ataxia and dysarthria in multiple sclerosis. *J Clin Neurosci* 2014;**21**:174–5.

Klaas JP, Burkholder DB, Singer W, Boes CJ. Harry Lee Parker and paroxysmal dysarthria and ataxia. *Neurology* 2013;**80**:311–4.

Li Y, Zeng C, Luo T. Paroxysmal dysarthria and ataxia in multiple sclerosis and corresponding magnetic resonance imaging findings. *J Neurol* 2011;**258**:273–6.

Marcel C, Anheim M, Flamand-Rouviere C, et al. Symptomatic paroxysmal dysarthria-ataxia in demyelinating diseases. *J Neurol* 2010;**257**:1369–72.

McArdle MJ. McArdle's sign in multiple sclerosis. *J Neurol Neurosurg Psychiatry* 1988;**51**:1110.

Darlix A, Mathey G, Sauvee M, Braun M, Debouverie M. Paroxysmal hypothermia in two patients with multiple sclerosis. *Eur Neurol* 2012;**67**:268–71.

Linker RA, Mohr A, Cepek L, Gold R, Prange H. Core hypothermia in multiple sclerosis: case report with magnetic resonance imaging localization of a thalamic lesion. *Mult Scler* 2006;**12**:112–5.

Weiss N, Hasboun D, Demeret S, et al. Paroxysmal hypothermia as a clinical feature of multiple sclerosis. *Neurology* 2009;**72**:193–5.

Chapter

4

Challenges in the therapeutic management of MS

The main therapeutic goals of immunomodulatory MS therapies are to reduce clinical relapses and the accumulation of new MRI lesions. MRI findings of encouraging therapeutic responses include a reduction in the development of new T2 lesions, gadolinium-enhancing T1 lesions and T1 hypointensities ("black holes"), as well as brain and spinal cord atrophy that may either accompany focal MS lesions or be diffuse. An additional goal is to reduce short-term relapse-related disability with a long-term promise (which continues to be controversial) of reducing long-term disability regardless of relapse- or progression-related etiology. Detailed clinical histories document the relapse rate prior to and following the initiation of MS therapies. Caution needs to be exercised, however, as patient recall may be incomplete. Clinicians need to be aware as well when initiating or switching MS therapies of the tendency for "regression to the mean" number of attacks, where patients with a prior high relapse rate, simply due to the nature of the disease, return to experience fewer "baseline" attacks even without altering the therapy they receive. Additionally, the natural history of RRMS suggests that MS patients will experience fewer attacks as they age.

Gauging improvement or stability in neurological impairment is achieved both from history and neurological examination. Assessing functional ambulatory limitations is often a key historical element. The clinician may assess functional ambulatory limitations by taking into account a patient's history indicating progressive disease. For example, in patients who previously walked miles in past years before the onset of leg dragging or gait ataxia, this impairment will be experienced increasingly earlier when ambulating.

MRI findings may inform the clinician of both prior and new inflammatory activity. This is evidenced by gadolinium-enhancing T1 lesions and the accumulation of new T2 lesions and chronic, non-gadolinium-enhancing T1 hypointensities ("black

holes"). Brain and spinal cord atrophy on MRI may also become apparent progressively over time. While an ideal interval for serial MRI evaluations is not defined, some physicians recommend every 12–24 months in "average" activity MS patients in order to assess radiological stability, worsening or improvement over time in relation to the patients' therapies. Some patients with highly active MS or those on natalizumab may require more frequent brain MRIs, especially to check for early development of progressive multifocal leukoencephalopathy (PML).

Certainly, if the goals of immunomodulatory or symptomatic therapy are being met, then no changes would be required unless there are significant problems with medication tolerability. This remains a challenge for all the immunomodulatory MS medications to varying degrees. A detailed evaluation of common and idiopathic side effects associated with the medication will be required and further switching of medications on the basis of adherence and tolerability may be needed.

Case 18: A young man with treatment-resistant MS who abuses tobacco

A 32-year-old gentleman developed Lhermitte symptoms and an ascending sensory myelopathy twelve months prior to presentation. Six months later, he developed gait ataxia and symptoms of a recurrent sensory myelopathy. Subsequent to this, he developed right-sided then left-sided optic neuritis. He was treated with a course of intravenous corticosteroids on one occasion but had not yet initiated any immunomodulatory MS medications. Serum JC virus antibodies were checked and were found to be positive. There was no family history of multiple sclerosis. The patient himself did not abuse illicit drugs but had smoked half a pack of cigarettes per day for the last eight years.

On neurological examination, mental status was normal. Cranial nerves were normal as was motor

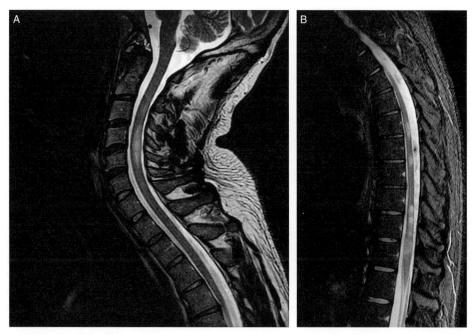

Figure 4.1 Sagittal T2 MRI cervical and thoracic spine showing multifocal T2 hyperintense lesions within the cervical and thoracic spinal cord compatible with multiple sclerosis.

examination. Reflexes were intact, with flexor plantar responses bilaterally and normal gait.

Brain and spinal cord MRI scans showed multiple areas of abnormal T2 hyperintense lesions consistent with multiple sclerosis (Figure 4.1). Repeated imaging showed resolved gadolinium enhancement in some of the lesions and also the development of new T2 lesions and many lesions that had new gadolinium enhancement. A CSF examination revealed elevated CSF oligoclonal bands.

Three-step assessment

1   Classical clinical features of MS: Lhermitte symptom, gait ataxia with resolution, recurrent inflammatory myelopathy, recurrent optic neuritis
2   Neurological examination: normal
3   Investigations: brain MRI consistent with MS; spinal cord MRI consistent with MS; CSF consistent with MS

Diagnosis: Relapsing-remitting multiple sclerosis with nicotine dependence.

Tip: It is critical to initiate immunomodulatory medications for patients with relapsing-remitting disease, particularly those with frequent relapses after onset of the disease as well as those who develop new MRI lesions early on. Such patients are more likely to

have more significant and more frequent attacks. In addition to this, it is imperative that these patients be encouraged to discontinue smoking immediately and offered the best medical assistance to do this. Patients who smoke cigarettes have difficulty controlling relapsing-remitting multiple sclerosis and have more challenging clinical courses according to most of the literature published on this question.

In this patient, despite the JC virus antibody positivity, it was considered that natalizumab still would be a possibility if its use was limited to 18 to 24 months, while the risk of developing progressive multifocal leukoencephalopathy (PML) is relatively low. Consideration of alternative immunomodulatory medications including interferons, fingolimod or dimethyl fumarate was also apt for this patient. He was directed to a nicotine-dependence clinic for nicotine cessation, which will be an important adjunct in his MS therapy.

Case 19:   A patient with continued relapses that is unresponsive to glatiramer acetate. Should she switch medications?

A 25-year-old woman awoke with binocular, painless, vertical and skewed diplopia that was worse on rightward gaze but which resolved spontaneously after a few weeks. Initially, an ophthalmologist diagnosed her with trochlear nerve palsy. On further consideration of her history, a Lhermitte symptom was identified earlier in the year of presentation. She had not had other symptoms that would suggest clinical features of attacks of multiple sclerosis apart from this. A paternal aunt was known to have multiple sclerosis, as was a distant maternal cousin. She was started on glatiramer acetate. She then had episodes consistent with three acute attacks of multiple sclerosis, including symptoms of an ascending cervical myelopathy, left-sided optic neuritis, and recurrent lower extremity numbness. She had been tolerating the glatiramer acetate well and had been adherent to it.

Her neurological examination was normal.

An initial brain MRI showed multiple areas of abnormal T2 signal, and one with gadolinium enhancement, consistent with multiple sclerosis. A repeat brain MRI showed an ongoing, active inflammatory component of her multiple sclerosis with many new gadolinium-enhancing lesions (Figure 4.2).

Three-step assessment

1 Classical clinical features of MS: painless binocular, diplopia recurrent inflammatory myelopathy, optic neuritis
2 Neurological examination: normal
3 Investigations: Brain MRI consistent with MS with activity

Diagnosis: Relapsing-remitting multiple sclerosis with activity, incomplete control of inflammation with glatiramer acetate.

The patient was switched to interferon beta 1a subcutaneously three times weekly. A repeat evaluation was performed. She had no new symptoms of clinical attacks over the next two years. Her neurological examination remained normal.

Tip: The two main indicators for switching MS therapies are tolerability and efficacy. This patient was adherent and tolerating glatiramer acetate but she continued to display ongoing clinical and radiological evidence of inflammation indicating incomplete efficacy. Clinicians must gauge the effectiveness of immunomodulatory medications of multiple sclerosis by estimating the prior and current relapse rate as well as new inflammatory MRI activity, and should change

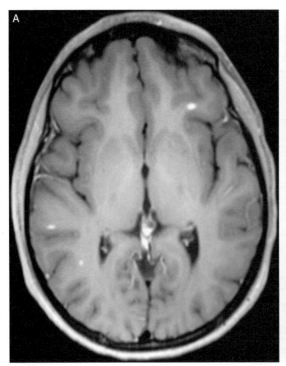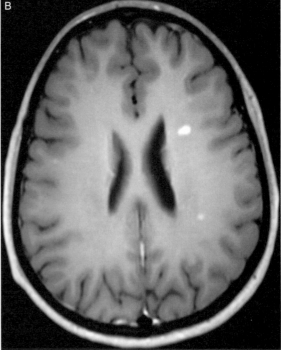

Figure 4.2 Axial T1 with gadolinium MRI brain showing substantial progression of multifocal contrast-enhancing lesions in the brain indicating incomplete control of the inflammatory component of MS.

immunomodulatory medications to reassess new effectiveness.

Case 20:   An MS patient intolerant of injections with bradycardia. What MS medications should be considered?

A 36-year-old gentleman was evaluated because of a history of right-sided foot dragging. Two months later it involved the right arm as well. He had not had prior episodes of clinical attacks and there was no family history of multiple sclerosis. He spontaneously improved, recovering to about 80 percent of normalcy without the use of steroids. The diagnosis was of a clinically isolated demyelination syndrome with a brainstem lesion. Multiple MRI MS lesions were found that put him at a high risk of developing relapsing-remitting multiple sclerosis. He initiated treatment with interferon beta 1a three times weekly but developed significant injection reaction pain so it was discontinued. The desire was to switch to an oral medication and fingolimod was identified as a major consideration. An electrocardiogram was done, which showed bradycardia at 46 beats per minute. His neurological examination was entirely normal.

A brain MRI scan showed areas of abnormal signal within the brainstem consistent with multiple sclerosis. A cervical spinal cord MRI showed T2 signal abnormality consistent with MS.

Three-step assessment
1   Classical clinical features of MS: brainstem attack; resolved hemiparesis
2   Neurological examination: normal
3   Investigations: brain MRI consistent with MS; spinal cord MRI consistent with MS

Diagnosis: Relapsing-remitting multiple sclerosis with injection intolerance.

Tip: The presented patient had therapeutic intolerance mainly related to injections. This would lessen the consideration of using other injectable medications such as other interferon preparations or glatiramer acetate. Fingolimod, generally speaking, should not be a strong consideration because of the significant bradycardia present. Bradycardia is worsened by the use of fingolimod, particularly the first dose due to its effects on sphingosine 1 –phosphate (S1P) receptors on the cardiac atrial muscle. First-dose monitoring for bradycardia

is recommended in all patients initiating treatment with fingolimod. Alternative oral MS therapies to be considered would be dimethyl fumarate or teriflunomide.

Case 21:   A woman with MS previously treated with natalizumab. Should natalizumab be reinitiated after progression on interferon therapy?

A 53-year-old woman presented for evaluation of treatment recommendations for multiple sclerosis. Approximately 21 years earlier she had symptoms of a sensory myelopathy that resolved with corticosteroids. She recalled having symptoms later that year of bilateral upper extremity numbness as well as right-sided optic neuritis, which did not improve. Her sister, cousin, and great aunt all had multiple sclerosis. She was initiated on interferon beta 1b every other day subcutaneously from 1995 for the next five years. She then changed to interferon beta 1a intramuscularly once weekly for the next 11 years.

She described a progressive impairment in her gait over the last 13 years. The patient required the use of a cane for the last 18 months. It was not clear that there had been any new definite clinical attacks or relapses in a number of years. She had worsened arm weakness after stress only. Because of the continued progressive worsening, she was changed to natalizumab one and a half years prior to being seen. She had received 15 infusions in total. The most recent evaluation for JC virus antibodies was six months prior to evaluation, and it remained negative.

On neurological examination, her mental status was found to be normal. She had mild weakness distally in the upper extremities and moderate weakness in a pyramidal distribution greater in the left than right lower extremity. She walked with a bilateral circumductive ataxic gait, and plantar responses were extensor bilaterally.

Repeat brain MRI scans revealed no new T2 lesions and no new gadolinium-enhancing lesions over many years of serial imaging. Repeat cervical and thoracic spine MRIs showed multiple chronic areas of demyelinating disease, again without evidence of new active demyelination or gadolinium enhancement. A JC virus serum antibody test was repeated and was now positive consistent with recent seroconversion.

Three-step assessment

1 Classical clinical features of MS: progressive quadriparetic gait disorder, optic neuritis; prior sensory myelopathy with resolution
2 Neurological examination: consistent with myelopathy
3 Investigations: brain MRI consistent with MS; spinal cord MRI consistent with MS

Diagnosis: Secondary progressive multiple sclerosis.

Tip: Check clinical history and imaging findings as well as old MRI reports to gauge whether there has been clear, new inflammatory activity consistent with relapsing forms of multiple sclerosis. If not, most immunomodulatory medications should not be strongly considered.

Given that this patient's gait had worsened over the last ten years and she had a 22-year disease course, it was suggestive that she has secondary progressive multiple sclerosis rather than a relapsing inflammatory component.

Repeat serological testing for JC virus-negative patients should take place approximately every six months to assess for seroconversion. In this patient, consideration was not made for natalizumab given the secondary progressive course. In addition to that, she is now JC virus antibody positive, which would put her at risk for progressive multifocal leukoencephalopathy (PML).

Case 22: Episodic symptomatic worsening in a patient with MS. Should highly aggressive immunomodulatory therapy be recommended?

A 62-year-old woman came for assessment. Her symptom onset began approximately three decades earlier. She had relapsing symptoms of vertigo or upper extremity weakness and numbness, always with resolution. Despite the onset and symptoms, she was evaluated formally for this only three years prior to evaluation. She recalls walking three or four miles a day dating back to five years prior to evaluation. She then started to require unilateral gait assistance three years prior to evaluation and started to use bilateral ski poles for one year prior to evaluation. A paternal aunt was known to have multiple sclerosis, and a sister had optic neuritis.

She initially was treated with glatiramer acetate but suffered from side effects. She was then started on dimethyl fumarate. She was hospitalized on four or five occasions prior to evaluation. She had symptomatic worsening: once with an influenza vaccination, once with a colonoscopy and once with angina pectoris. The patient reported that after the hospitalizations, she was essentially wheelchair bound but had recovered enough so that she could walk on occasion with her ski poles for about one block only.

She had no new symptoms of spontaneous clinical attacks of multiple sclerosis such as optic neuritis, new-onset diplopia, dysarthria, hemiparesis or hemisensory deficit.

On neurological examination she had a moderate upper motor neuron pattern quadriparesis with spasticity and a right greater than left circumductive gait impairment. Plantar response was extensor on the right and flexor on the left. She had vibratory sensory loss in the feet bilaterally.

Serial brain and spinal cord MRI scans showed no evidence of new inflammatory multiple sclerosis lesions even during times of symptomatic worsening (Figure 4.3).

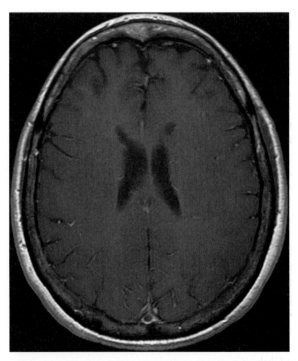

Figure 4.3 Axial T1 MRI brain showing an ovoid chronic and inactive area of T1 hypointensity ("black hole") consistent with chronic MS. Cervical and thoracic spine MRIs showed multifocal, non-enhancing T2 hyperintense lesions (not shown). Pseudoexacerbations are common in patients with progressive forms of MS.

Three-step assessment

1 Classical clinical features of MS: relapsing limb numbness and weakness, progressive cervical myelopathy
2 Neurological examination: upper motor neuron quadriparesis
3 Investigations: brain MRI consistent with MS; spinal cord MRI consistent with MS

Diagnosis: Pseudoexacerbations of multiple sclerosis.

Tip: Pseudoexacerbations of multiple sclerosis can be associated with severe impairment. They are often identifiable by accompanying conditions such as infections, elevated body temperature, fatigue and others in patients with progressive MS clinical courses (primary and secondary progressive MS). Repeat neuroimaging can be helpful in assessing whether there is any new inflammatory activity if there is uncertainty in discriminating between relapsing and progressive disease and in determining whether impairment may be due exclusively to pseudoexacerbations. Natalizumab should not be recommended as it is not approved for secondary progressive multiple sclerosis.

Case 23: An MS patient considering pregnancy. When should medications be initiated or stopped?

A 34-year-old woman presented with right optic neuritis ten years ago. A CSF examination was inconclusive. Months later, she developed symptoms of a sensory myelopathy with resolution. Brain and cervical spine MRI scans showed typical brain MS lesions and a short-segment spinal cord T2 lesion consistent with MS. Serum NMO-IgG antibodies were negative. She initiated treatment with interferon beta -1a subcutaneously three times weekly.

She had been off and on that interferon because of intervening family planning. She described injection site reactions and flu-like symptoms that were resistant to the use of acetaminophen. She considered glatiramer acetate but did not want to go on long-standing injections. No medications were delivered for the last 20 months. She runs 20 miles per week without difficulty, but occasionally experiences a Uhthoff phenomenon in the right eye with exercise.

Her neurological examination was normal.

Three-step assessment

1 Classical clinical features of MS: optic neuritis, Uhthoff phenomenon; acute sensory myelopathy
2 Neurological examination: normal
3 Investigations: brain MRI consistent with MS; spinal cord MRI consistent with MS; CSF inconclusive

Diagnosis: Currently relatively benign multiple sclerosis.

Tip: Reviewing both the goals of immunomodulatory therapy and reduction of clinical attacks in new MRI lesions of MS in addition to that of family planning is critical when making a decision. Glatiramer acetate is a pregnancy category B medication and some observational reports suggest pregnancies occurring with its use are safe. Teriflunomide is a pregnancy category X medication with teratogenic findings in animal studies. It is generally recommended currently that all immunomodulatory medications be discontinued approximately three months prior to attempting to conceive a child and throughout breast feeding. They can be reinitiated following delivery of the baby and completion of breastfeeding if desired.

Case 24: An MS patient with psoriasis on interferon beta 1a three times weekly with incomplete efficacy. Which alternative oral MS therapy should be used?

This patient had multiple sclerosis with ongoing relapses, including most recently hand and leg numbness (left greater than right) associated with a Lhermitte symptom and worsening imbalance. He was treated with interferon beta 1a three times weekly and was both tolerant and adherent to interferon therapy. He was previously treated with glatiramer acetate with incomplete response to the inflammatory component of his disease. He had a long history of psoriasis but had never been treated with tumor necrosis factor (TNF) alpha antagonists.

On neurological examination, his mental status was found to be normal, as were extraocular movements with no internuclear ophthalmoplegia. Motor power was normal throughout with an extensor right plantar response. His gait was ataxic.

Repeat brain MRI scans showed multiple areas of abnormal signal, a number with gadolinium enhancement. There were new areas of abnormal signal on T2-weighted imaging of the spinal cord and subtle enhancement on a couple of lesions there as well.

Three-step assessment

1 Classical clinical features of MS: recurrent upper and lower extremity numbness with Lhermitte symptom, gait ataxia
2 Neurological examination: normal
3 Investigations: brain MRI consistent with MS; spinal cord MRI consistent with MS

Diagnosis: Relapsing-remitting multiple sclerosis with activity, incomplete response to interferon therapy and glatiramer acetate therapy.

Tip: Since this patient had new inflammatory myelopathy and neuroimaging evidence of an ongoing inflammatory process despite the interferons, he was counseled that a switch to an alternative immunomodulatory medication was necessary. JC virus antibody testing was checked and found to be negative, indicating no definite prior exposure to the JC virus and a low risk of developing progressive multifocal leukoencephalopathy (PML). He considered the use of dimethyl fumarate as an alternative; dimethyl fumarate was developed from a fumaric acid drug used for psoriasis. It should be noted that rare psoriasis patients treated with fumaric acid esters have developed PML. The dimethyl fumarate might have a salutary effect on the psoriasis as a secondary gain. Natalizumab would be a reasonable infusion-based MS therapy as an alternative given the current JC virus seronegative result.

Case 25: A woman with MS is investigated for vascular abnormalities

A 20-year-old woman initially presented with right arm and leg numbness that progressed over a number of days. There was no definite weakness and no facial involvement initially. She had a Lhermitte symptom. The sensory symptoms lasted for four months and then resolved spontaneously without treatment with corticosteroids. Brain and spinal cord MRI scans showed changes highly suggestive of multiple sclerosis.

At the recommendation of a friend, she sought vascular imaging in Canada. An MR venography of the brain and neck were interpreted to be normal. A neck ultrasound showed evidence of one of the "Zamboni criteria" with reflux involving the right internal jugular vein and in an upright position only. The azygous vein was not well seen on MR venography, but it was felt that could be due to hypoplasia.

The patient then travelled to Costa Rica for treatment of suspected chronic cerebrospinal venous insufficiency (CCSVI). Angioplasties of the right and left internal jugular veins as well as the azygous vein were performed without stenting. She experienced some symptomatic improvement in mental fogginess, but the symptoms returned six months later.

She then developed new onset numbness and tingling from the chest down consistent with a spinal cord sensory level. Repeat neuroimaging showed multiple areas of new abnormal MRI signal, many with gadolinium enhancement consistent with active MS. She altered her diet but did not initiate immunomodulatory medications.

On neurological examination, she had significant gait imbalance with left lower extremity upper motor neuron pattern weakness with a left extensor plantar response. She had mild vibratory sensory loss in the feet bilaterally.

Repeat brain and cervical spine MRI scans showed multiple areas of abnormal signals consistent with highly active multiple sclerosis (Figure 4.4). A CSF examination showed elevated oligoclonal bands and an elevated IgG index.

Three-step assessment

1 Classical clinical features of MS: recurrent sensory myelopathy with Lhermitte symptom, gait ataxia
2 Neurological examination: left upper motor neuron type weakness gait ataxia and distal vibratory sense loss
3 Investigations: brain MRI consistent with MS; spinal cord MRI consistent with MS; CSF examination consistent with MS

Diagnosis: Relapsing-remitting multiple sclerosis with untreated marked inflammatory disease.

Tip: Cerebrospinal venous abnormalities are not associated with multiple sclerosis, may delay appropriate MS therapy and encourage unnecessary and potentially harmful vascular procedures. The findings of CCSVI by Zamboni and colleagues in Italy have not been confirmed independently by other researchers to have diagnostic or therapeutic significance in MS.

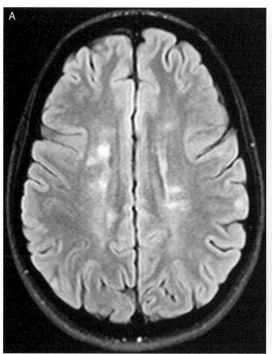
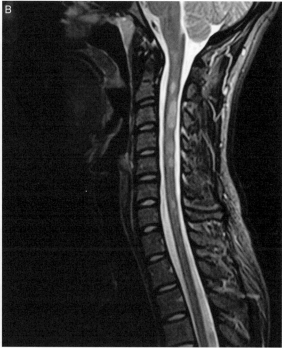

Figure 4.4 A) Axial FLAIR MRI brain with callosal, periventricular and juxtacortical T2 MS lesions. B) Sagittal T2 MRI cervical spinal cord showing multifocal T2 hyperintense lesions compatible with multiple sclerosis.

Case 26 An MS patient with acute right lower extremity pain. Is it due to established MS?

A 46-year-old gentleman had a clear history of multiple sclerosis dating back two decades. At that time, he had typical symptoms of a sensory myelopathy and optic neuritis. He had formally been diagnosed with multiple sclerosis 22 years prior to evaluation and had approximately five or six clinical attacks of multiple sclerosis, at one time developing severe left optic neuritis and gait impairment.

He had been on immunomodulatory medications with various interferon preparations and, because of gait impairment, was started on dalfampridine. He suffered slowly progressive impairment in the lower extremities with weakness without bowel and bladder impairment.

About three years prior to presentation, while walking around a grocery store, he had a sudden onset of severe pain and weakness involving the left lower extremity. Since that time, he was hospitalized for chronic pain and required narcotic analgesics. He did not have a significant allodynic type of pain, and

he experienced some pain with spasms as well. He had received corticosteroids without improvement in his motor weakness. He then underwent plasma exchange for steroid-unresponsive impairment. He completed four plasma exchanges without improvement.

On neurological examination he was found to be drowsy, likely due to narcotic pain medication. His cranial nerve exam was normal. An upper extremity exam revealed normal tone, power and coordination. He had upper motor neuron pattern weakness bilaterally in the lower extremity with less movement of the left lower extremity. His deep tendon reflexes were globally brisk in the upper and lower extremities, with the left plantar response being flexor, the right extensor. On manipulating the left lower extremity, he had considerable tenderness below the knee, in the calf.

In repeat brain, cervical and thoracic spine MRI scans, multiple areas of abnormal T2 signal consistent with chronic demyelination were found without gadolinium enhancement (Figure 4.5). An EMG study showed multiple but inactive left lower extremity radiculopathies and poor motor unit activation consistent with a central nervous system disorder.

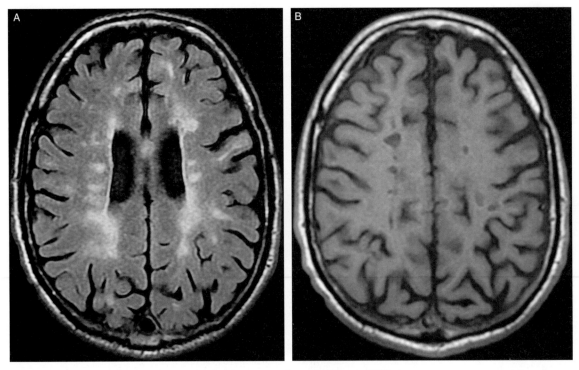

Figure 4.5 Axial FLAIR and T1 MRI brain with callosal, periventricular and juxtacortical MS lesions.

On routine evaluation by a physical therapist while hospitalized for plasma exchange, the left lower extremity was measured and found to be shorter than the right. There was pain experienced on passive range of motion in the left hip. Hip x-rays showed an old subcapital fracture with femoral avascular hip necrosis (Figure 4.6). He underwent a hip arthroplasty with marked improvement in pain control.

Three-step assessment

1 Classical clinical features of MS: recurrent myelopathy, optic neuritis, progressive myelopathy
2 Neurological examination: lower extremity upper motor neuron type weakness with pain in left lower extremity
3 Investigations: brain MRI consistent with MS; spinal cord MRI consistent with MS; EMG chronic radicular changes without activity; hip x-ray left avascular hip necrosis with subcapital femoral fracture

 Diagnosis: Secondary Progressive MS with hip fracture from avascular hip necrosis.

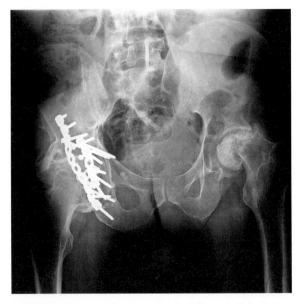

Figure 4.6 Hip x-ray showing subcapital fracture of the left femoral neck with sclerosis and fragmentation of the left femoral head suggesting avascular hip necrosis. Posttraumatic deformity of the right acetabulum with screw and plate fixation is also shown.

Tip: Look for joint causes of atypical types of pain in patients with chronic multiple sclerosis. Measuring the legs is beneficial when looking for hip fractures. Avascular hip necrosis can occur with the use of corticosteroids used typically for attacks of multiple sclerosis. Plasma exchange is not found to be beneficial for patients with old and inactive or progressive forms of multiple sclerosis. It is used for rescue therapy for recent, corticosteroid unresponsive, CNS inflammatory demyelinating attacks with severe functional impairment only.

Further reading

Fox RJ, Miller DH, Phillips JT, et al. Placebo-controlled phase 3 study of oral BG-12 or glatiramer in multiple sclerosis. *The New England Journal of Medicine* 2012;**367**: 1087–97.

Pelletier D, Hafler DA. Fingolimod for multiple sclerosis. *The New England Journal of Medicine* 2012;**366**: 339–47.

Dorr J, Paul F. The transition from first-line to second-line therapy in multiple sclerosis. *Curr Treat Options Neurol* 2015;**17**:354.

Freedman MS, Abdoli M. Evaluating response to disease-modifying therapy in relapsing multiple sclerosis. *Expert Rev Neurother* 2015;**15**:407–23.

Goodin DS. The use of interferon Beta and glatiramer acetate in multiple sclerosis. *Semin Neurol* 2013;**33**:13–25.

Lublin FD, Cofield SS, Cutter GR, et al. Randomized study combining interferon and glatiramer acetate in multiple sclerosis. *Ann Neurol* 2013;**73**:327–40.

Willis MA, Cohen JA. Fingolimod therapy for multiple sclerosis. *Semin Neurol* 2013;**33**:37–44.

Bourdette DN, Cohen JA. Venous angioplasty for "CCSVI" in multiple sclerosis: ending a therapeutic misadventure. *Neurology* 2014;**83**:388–9.

Carruthers RL, Berger J. Progressive multifocal leukoencephalopathy and JC Virus-related disease in modern neurology practice. *Mult Scler Relat Disord* 2014;**3**:419–30.

Correale J, Farez MF. Smoking worsens multiple sclerosis prognosis: Two different pathways are involved. *J Neuroimmunol* 2015;**281**:23–34.

Manouchehrinia A, Weston M, Tench CR, Britton J, Constantinescu CS. Tobacco smoking and excess mortality in multiple sclerosis: a cohort study. *J Neurol Neurosurg Psychiatry* 2014;**85**:1091–5.

Salzer J, Hallmans G, Nystrom M, Stenlund H, Wadell G, Sundstrom P. Smoking as a risk factor for multiple sclerosis. *Mult Scler* 2013;**19**:1022–7.

Siddiqui AH, Zivadinov R, Benedict RH, et al. Prospective randomized trial of venous angioplasty in MS (PREMiSe). *Neurology* 2014;**83**:441–9.

Traboulsee AL, Knox KB, Machan L, et al. Prevalence of extracranial venous narrowing on catheter venography in people with multiple sclerosis, their siblings, and unrelated healthy controls: a blinded, case-control study. *Lancet* 2014;**383**:138–45.

Tur C, Montalban X. Natalizumab: risk stratification of individual patients with multiple sclerosis. *CNS Drugs* 2014;**28**:641–8.

Wingerchuk DM. Smoking: effects on multiple sclerosis susceptibility and disease progression. *Ther Adv Neurol Disord* 2012;**5**:13–22.

Xu Z, Zhang F, Sun F, Gu K, Dong S, He D. Dimethyl fumarate for multiple sclerosis. *Cochrane Database Syst Rev* 2015;**4**:CD011076.

Challenges in diagnosing demyelinating ocular disease

Introduction

Visual impairment is common in multiple sclerosis and is usually due to optic neuritis. As previously described, this is typically a painful unilateral visual impairment that worsens over hours to days, then improves over days to weeks with excellent, but often incomplete, resolution. Painless, binocular, vertical, horizontal or oblique diplopia and, less commonly, oscillopsia (perception of movement of the visual background with body or head motion) and hemianopia may also occur with MS. Pitfalls may occur in assessing visual disorders related to, and possibly associated with, multiple sclerosis.

Case 27: A history of visual disturbance in a young woman. Is it due to MS?

A 39-year-old woman noticed a disturbance in her vision two years prior to assessment. The onset was uncertain and initially the disturbance was attributed to color vision impairment, which bothered her while driving, but she could not reliably describe what the visual problem was. She described difficulty discriminating "where the area was that she was supposed to drive." Months later, she had a painless central visual loss over two weeks that responded to corticosteroid treatment. The latter visual impairment was associated with Uhthoff phenomenon which worsened with exercise and high body temperature, and progressive visual loss as the day went on that was worsened by high humidity and high ambient temperatures. She had no prior symptoms of visual loss more typical of painful optic neuritis.

She denied having prior diplopia, dysarthria or dysphagia, hearing loss or ptosis. She had not experienced a Lhermitte symptom, nor hemiparesis, hemisensory deficit or symptoms of sensory myelopathy, and her ambulation was entirely unrestricted. There was no family history of multiple sclerosis.

On neurological examination, visual fields were entirely full with a visual acuity of 20/40 in the right eye and 20/100 in the left eye, which did not improve on evaluation with a pinhole (indicating that the acuity impairment was not due to refractive error). Her optic discs were pale bilaterally and she had impaired color vision in both eyes. Extraocular movements revealed right greater than left incomplete, bilateral internuclear ophthalmoplegia. Her motor exam was normal with bilateral extensor plantar responses.

Three-step assessment

1 Classical clinical features of MS: Uhthoff phenomenon, painless optic neuropathy
2 Neurological examination consistent with MS: optic neuropathies with bilateral internuclear ophthalmoplegia and extensor plantar responses
3 Investigations: MRI brain consistent with MS

Diagnosis: Relapsing-remitting multiple sclerosis.

Tip: Patients with internuclear ophthalmoplegia often do not complain of distinct diplopia. Their symptoms are often rather nonspecific, as they were in this case. The examination finding of bilateral internuclear ophthalmoplegia is highly suggestive of multiple sclerosis as the cause. Internuclear ophthalmoplegia is best diagnosed clinically by having the patient make rapid horizontal saccades from the extreme left to the extreme right repeatedly to elicit slowed medial adduction and accompanying dysconjugate nystagmus of the abducting eye, which is consistent with incomplete internuclear ophthalmoplegia. The Uhthoff phenomenon of impaired and graying out vision is consistent with prior demyelinating optic neuropathies. This is due to a conduction block with an increased body temperature.

Case 28: A patient with optic atrophy and abnormal brain MRI scan. Is it MS? Should immunomodulatory medications be used?

A 47-year-old woman presented ten years earlier with sudden, painless visual loss involving the left eye's superior and temporal visual fields but with preserved central vision. The right eye was entirely normal. An ophthalmologist reportedly found evidence of an optic nerve head edema with normal ocular pressures and diagnosed her with optic neuritis. She was treated with corticosteroids which led to some improvement in her vision over the next three to four weeks, and she was almost entirely back to normal after six months. The following year she awoke with a headache and noticed some "spots" in the right eye associated with a pressure sensation. Again she was treated with corticosteroids.

She had no prior classical MS symptoms such as diplopia, dysarthria, dysphagia, hemiparesis or hemi-sensory deficit. She did not have a Lhermitte symptom. She had mild tinnitus but no hearing loss. Ambulation was entirely unrestricted. She had a history of cigarette smoking and marijuana use with a remote history of alcohol overuse but that was in remission. The clinical suspicion at that time was that she had multiple sclerosis, and she initiated treatment with interferon beta 1a intramuscular once weekly.

Her mental status and cranial nerves were normal. Visual fields were full to confrontation, while her optic discs appeared normal. There was no relative afferent pupillary defect. Color vision was normal. Extraocular movements were full and normal without internuclear ophthalmoplegia. Her motor exam was normal with brisk but symmetrical reflexes and flexor plantar responses. Her gait and sensory examinations were normal.

Her brain MRI results were atypical for demyelinating disease but more consistent with small vessel ischemic changes. A CSF examination showed normal results without elevations in unique CSF oligoclonal bands or IgG index. Visual evoked potentials were normal. Serological evaluations, including a complete blood count, erythrocyte sedimentation rate, vitamin B12, Lyme serology and a paraneoplastic autoantibody screen, were normal.

A watchful waiting approach was initiated. Follow-ups took place every two years for the next ten years and she had no further symptoms and no

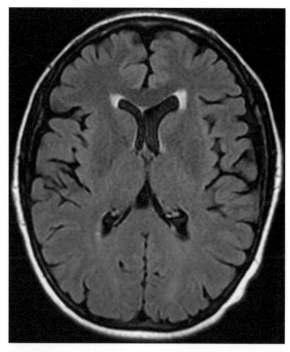

Figure 5.1 Axial FLAIR MRI brain showed several scattered foci of T2 hyperintensity in the white matter that were nonspecific in appearance and unchanged over 8 years of follow-up.

change in her ocular evaluation. Repeat serial brain scans showed no development of typical MS lesions (Figure 5.1).

Three-step assessment

1 Classical clinical features of MS: monocular, painless visual loss, uncertain optic neuritis
2 Neurological examination: normal without significant optic neuropathy
3 Investigations: MRI brain not consistent with MS; CSF not consistent with MS; visual evoked potentials normal; follow-up not consistent with MS

Diagnosis: Visual loss, no definite MS diagnosis.

Tip: A watchful waiting approach is sometimes extremely beneficial when the diagnosis of multiple sclerosis remains uncertain. Repeating clinical and radiological evaluations over time to assess for the development of more definitive changes of multiple sclerosis is important. Avoiding directed immunomodulatory therapy aimed at MS is important where diagnostic uncertainty remains. The patient had no dissemination of symptoms, non-specific MRI findings and a normal CSF over ten years of follow-up not meeting MS criteria.

Case 29: Is it papillitis (optic neuritis) or papilledema?

A 36-year-old gentleman was found to have a bilateral optic nerve head edema of uncertain etiology.

The patient was aware of visual symptoms for one and a half months. He described episodes of his vision "fading out," where his visual fields would constrict from the periphery inward from both eyes simultaneously. On some occasions only the extreme peripheral vision would darken and at other times his vision bilaterally would be lost completely. The visual impairment would last less than ten minutes with the vision then resolving entirely back to normal. Leaning his head and body forward and turning his head to one side could initiate the visual disturbance. The visual symptoms were not associated with seeing scintillating scotoma, waves, jagged edges or fortification spectra, and he had no ptosis or diplopia. He had no headache or pulsatile tinnitus and had no prior symptoms of hemiparesis, hemisensory deficit or loss of consciousness, and even during the spells his mental status remained entirely normal. He had a sedentary lifestyle and had gained 40 pounds of weight over the prior year.

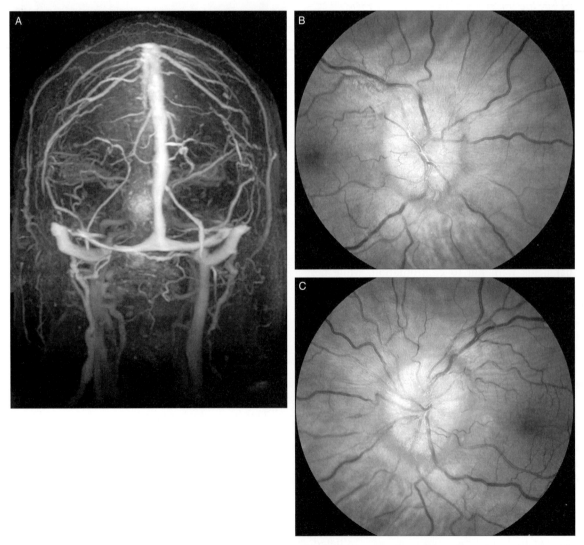

Figure 5.2 A) MR Venography showed both transverse sinuses were narrowed without evidence of thrombosis. This can be seen with idiopathic intracranial hypertension. An MRI brain scan showed no evidence of intracranial mass lesions. B,C) An ophthalmological examination showed a bilateral disc edema; a lumbar puncture opening pressure was 420 mm H20.

On neurological examination, visual acuity was 20/20 in the right eye and 20/20–1 in the left eye with normal color vision bilaterally and no afferent pupillary defect. Intraocular pressures were normal bilaterally. A dilated funduscopy showed an optic nerve head edema with small flame hemorrhages extending beyond the optic nerve in both eyes (Figure 5.2 B,C). Retinal periphery was normal. The rest of his neurological examination was normal.

A brain MRI scan did not show any intracranial mass lesions or other signal abnormality of significance but showed radiological evidence of bilateral papilledema with dilatation of the optic nerve sheaths. MR venography showed no evidence of venous thrombosis but the transverse sinuses were narrowed bilaterally (Figure 5.2 A). A CSF examination was normal apart from the documented opening CSF pressure of 42 cm of H_2O. Serological testing excluded syphilis, ehrlichia and Lyme disease as the possible cause.

Three-step assessment

1 Classical clinical features of MS: visual symptoms atypical for optic neuritis (positional, bilateral, transient, painless visual obscurations of brief duration)
2 Neurological examination: optic nerve head edema bilaterally without acuity loss or color vision impairment
3 Investigations: MRI brain not consistent with MS; CSF not consistent with MS with elevated opening CSF pressure

Diagnosis: Idiopathic intracranial hypertension (pseudotumor cerebri).

Tip: an enlarged optic nerve head due to "papillitis," that is, optic neuritis is typically associated with severe loss of visual acuity and color vision impairment. Papilledema from increased intracranial pressure may be associated with transient visual obscurations, as in this patient, as well as enlargement of the physiological blind spot but unless this is extremely severe, it is less likely to cause visual acuity deficit despite the marked optic nerve head edema seen.

A brain MRI scan ruled out demyelinating lesions of MS and any significant intracranial mass lesion. An MR venography ruled out any significant sinus venous thrombosis, which can cause a similar picture. Documentation of definitive elevated CSF opening pressure, as was performed in this case, is essential in making the diagnosis of pseudotumor cerebri.

The patient was started on acetazolamide 500 mg by mouth twice daily. This may have an effect on carbonic anhydrase inhibition to reduce CSF pressure. It also may cause reduced appetite, and be associated with beneficial weight loss.

Case 30: An elderly woman presenting with rapid and severe bilateral visual loss

A 78-year-old woman presented with a nine-day history of progressive, severe, bilateral and painless visual loss, essentially equivalent in the right and left eyes. She rapidly became functionally blind over the two days prior to presentation. She had no prior history of visual loss and had no history of diplopia, hemiparesis, hemisensory deficit, symptoms of sensory myelopathy, gait impairment or bowel or bladder dysfunction.

On neurological examination it was found that she had severe, bilateral blindness with poorly responsive pupils without any optic nerve head edema (papilledema). The rest of her neurological examination was normal.

A brain MRI showed a gadolinium-enhancing lesion involving both optic nerves and the optic chiasm (Figure 5.3). Age-appropriate small vessel ischemic changes were seen in the brain's white matter but none were suggestive of MS. A CSF examination showed no unique oligoclonal bands or elevated IgG index. Serum paraneoplastic autoantibodies were negative. Serum SS-B antibodies were minimally elevated but a salivary gland biopsy showed no diagnostic features of Sjögren syndrome. Serum NMO-IgG (aquaporin-4) antibodies were positive.

She was treated with 1000 mg of intravenous methylprednisolone for five days. She was started on treatment with azathioprine after serum thiopurine methyltransferase (TPMT) enzyme level assessment was found to be adequate. She experienced marked improvement with good functional vision regained. She remained on chronic immunosuppressive medications to reduce the likelihood of recurrent NMO spectrum disorder attacks even following a single clinical attack.

Three-step assessment

1 Classical clinical features of MS: acute optic neuropathies, atypical for MS-related optic neuritis (very severe, painless and bilateral at onset)

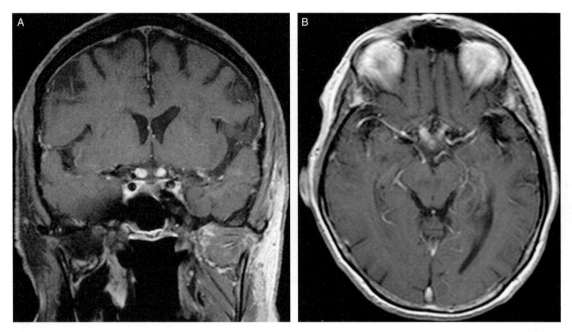

Figure 5.3 Coronal and Axial T1 with gadolinium MRI brain and optic nerves shows marked gadolinium enhancement of the posterior optic nerves and into the optic chiasm.

2 Neurological examination: severe bilateral optic neuropathies

3 Investigations: MRI brain not consistent with MS with optic chiasm involvement; CSF not consistent with MS; NMO-IGG antibody positive

   Diagnosis: Bilateral severe optic neuritis related to neuromyelitis optica (NMO) spectrum disease.

   Tip: Optic nerve and optic chiasmal lesions with severe optic neuropathies, particularly bilaterally, can suggest neuromyelitis optica spectrum disease. Patients with elevated NMO-IgG antibodies are at higher risk of developing new clinical attacks of neuromyelitis optica and so should be considered strongly for the use of long-term immunosuppressive medications.

Case 31: A young woman with headaches, optic nerve head edema and abnormal brain MRI

A 33-year-old woman with a history of migraine and rheumatoid arthritis on no medications presented with a three-week history of new onset visual symptoms. She described "floaters" in her right eye which then went on to involve the left eye, which were constantly present and progressively spread throughout her vision. On some occasions she had seconds where her vision seemed "all fuzzy" all over, and this progressed to a point where she had had difficulty reading and seeing a computer screen. She had had moderate headaches that had worsened over the prior three weeks. She had mild gait imbalance and felt nonspecific weakness in her legs and rare spells of paresthesias in random distributions. She had no fever or contact with sick people, and did not travel to a significant degree. She had had some intermittent spells of paresthesias in different distributions.

She was evaluated in ophthalmology where she was found to have visual acuity of 20/100 in the right eye and 20/100 in the left eye with bilateral optic disk edema, macular edema and exudates and blot hemorrhages (Figure 5.4).

On neurological evaluation her mental status was normal. Motor and sensory examination was normal. Her reflexes were symmetric and normal with flexor plantar responses. There was no limb or gait ataxia.

Nursing completed vital signs at admission and found the patient's arterial blood pressure was 263/164 mm Hg with consistent elevation on repeated testing.

A brain MRI showed diffuse increased T2 signal involving the bilateral cerebral hemispheres, with extensive white matter involvement especially periventricular, cerebellar hemispheres and significant involvement of the brainstem (Figure 5.5). There was some minimal perivascular gadolinium enhancement. A spinal cord MRI showed nonspecific, diffuse, patchy segmental T2 signal abnormality throughout the cervical and thoracic cord with subtle contrast enhancement. A CSF examination demonstrated normal CSF opening pressure, 9 white blood cells, 65 red blood cells with a markedly elevated protein at 165 mg/dL, no xanthochromia and normal glucose. Tests for Bartonella, histoplasma, Lyme, HIV, cytomegalovirus, herpes simplex virus, JC virus, and West Nile virus were negative. Oligoclonal bands were negative and her IgG index was normal.

Three-step assessment

1 Classical clinical features of MS: visual disorder atypical for optic neuritis
2 Neurological examination: visual acuity loss with optic nerve edema, with profound retinal vascular changes; extremely high blood pressure
3 Investigations: MRI brain not consistent with MS; MRI spinal cord not consistent with MS; CSF not consistent with MS

Diagnosis: Malignant hypertension with leukoencephalopathy and bilateral optic neuropathies.

Tip: Patients with bilateral optic nerve head edema should have their blood pressure carefully evaluated. The MRI findings were far more severe than the clinical symptomatology in this patient and if the findings were due to a demyelinating cause, a devastating neurological presentation would be expected. With maintenance of strict blood pressure control the MRI abnormalities and clinical symptoms resolved. No definite secondary cause for malignant hypertension was found in this patient.

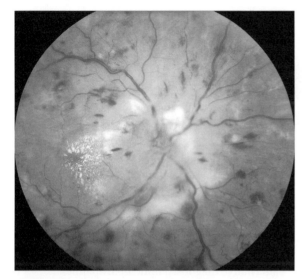

Figure 5.4 Fundus photography of the right eye shows severe disc edema with prominent macular exudates, areas of retinal whitening and a combination of flame-shaped and dot-blot hemorrhages scattered throughout the posterior pole.

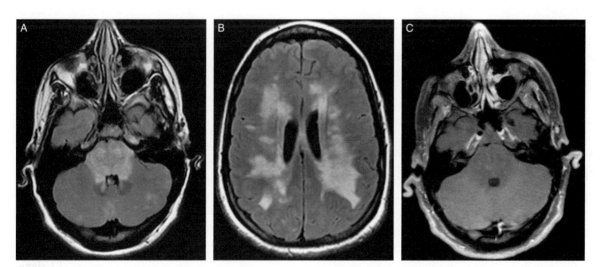

Figure 5.5 Axial FLAIR and T1 with gadolinium MRI brain showing Florid T2 signal abnormality involving the periventricular white matter, deep white matter, entire brainstem and both cerebellar hemispheres. Lesions in the brainstem demonstrate punctate or stippled post gadolinium contrast enhancement.

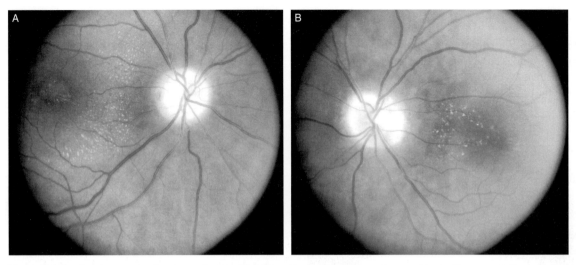

Figure 5.6 Fundus photography showing optic pallor bilaterally with macular star formation consistent with neuroretinitis.

Case 32: A young woman with recurrent visual loss and recurrent optic nerve head edema

A 34-year-old woman had a long history of visual impairment. About 15 years previously, she had headaches and right-sided ocular pain associated with visual blurriness. An ophthalmological examination revealed right-sided optic nerve head edema.

Over the following ten years, she had recurrent symptoms of visual impairment accompanied by optic nerve head edema first involving the right eye and then involving the left eye along with significant visual acuity impairment. She was treated on numerous occasions with intravenous methylprednisolone and oral prednisone and acetazolamide.

A neurological examination showed waxing and waning optic nerve head edema in the affected eye with macular stars and subsequent bilateral optic atrophy (Figure 5.6). The rest of her neurological examination was normal.

Repeated brain and spinal cord MRI scans were normal without evidence of MS. Repeated CSF examinations did not show elevated oligoclonal bands or IgG index and CSF opening pressures were normal. Vitamin B12 antinuclear antibodies, hemoglobin A1 C, lactate, phospholipid antibodies and a paraneoplastic screen were negative. Lyme disease, leptospirosis, toxoplasmosis and acute Epstein-Barr virus infections were all excluded.

Three-step assessment

1 Classical clinical features of MS: recurrent optic neuropathies
2 Neurological examination: consistent with alternative diagnosis; optic neuropathies consistently with optic nerve head edema; macular star formation consistent with neuroretinitis
3 Investigations: MRI brain not consistent with MS; MRI spinal cord not consistent with MS; CSF not consistent with MS

Diagnosis: Relapsing neuroretinitis, presumably autoimmune.

Tip: Neuroretinitis was described by Leber in 1916 as a stellate maculopathy. An important feature of an optic neuropathy is that it is often painless, although discomfort can occur. A macular star figure may occur, which consists of lipid or hard exudates occurring within days to weeks after visual impairment. This becomes more prominent as the optic nerve head edema resolves. Infectious etiologies and malignant hypertension need to be ruled out as possibilities. The macular star often resolves after 6–12 months. A recurrent idiopathic form of neuroretinitis possibly representing an autoimmune vasculitis of the disc exists without any apparent increased risk for multiple sclerosis.

Case 33: A man with visual loss, optic nerve head edema and an abnormal chest x-ray

A 50-year-old man presented with a history of headache and scotoma involving the right eye. He was treated initially with intravenous methyl-prednisolone and prednisone, then with intravenous immunoglobulin with no early benefit, but vision returned to normal in one year. Three years later, a recurrent "washed-out" sensation of the left eye occurred and optic nerve head edema was again found. Bilateral Uhthoff phenomenon was present.

The patient had no previous symptoms of multiple sclerosis attacks, and there was no family history of multiple sclerosis or other neurological disease. He was a nonsmoker with no constitutional symptoms.

A neurological examination showed visual acuity of 20/40 in the right eye and 20/20 in the left eye. He had an otherwise normal neurological examination.

A brain MRI was found to be normal. A CSF examination showed twenty white blood cells and elevated oligoclonal bands. A repeat CSF examination

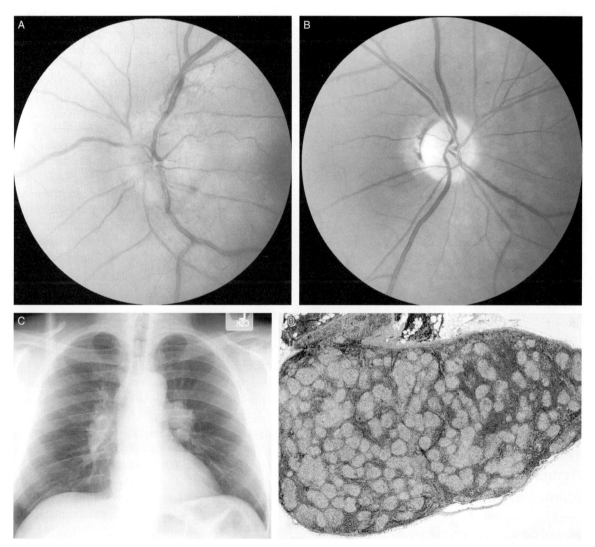

Figure 5.7 A, B): Fundus photography showing optic atrophy in the right eye with optic nerve head edema in the left eye. C) Chest x-ray shows bilateral hilar adenopathy, right greater than left; chest CT (not shown) demonstrated moderate adenopathy in mediastinum with small scattered bilateral pulmonary nodules consistent with pulmonary sarcoidosis. D) A biopsy specimen following mediastinoscopy demonstrated non-necrotizing granulomatous inflammation lower paratracheal lymph nodes consistent with sarcoidosis.

showed 31 white blood cells, negative oligoclonal bands, a normal IgG index and a mild protein elevation. Serological evaluations ruled out Lyme disease, syphilis and Bartonella. NMO-IgG antibodies were negative, as was serum angiotensin-converting enzyme (ACE). A chest x-ray showed bilateral hilar adenopathy that was greater on the left side with moderate mediastinal adenopathy with small pulmonary nodules (Figure 5.7). A bronchoscopy with biopsy was negative for malignancy and granulomas. A mediastinoscopy with biopsy showed evidence of nonnecrotizing granulomatous inflammation in the lower peritracheal lymph nodes.

Three-step assessment

1 Classical clinical features of MS: recurrent optic neuropathies
2 Neurological examination: consistent with alternative diagnosis: optic neuropathies with optic nerve head edema
3 Investigations: MRI brain not consistent with MS; CSF initially consistent with MS but then negative oligoclonal bands; chest imaging and pathology consistent with sarcoidosis

Diagnosis: Neurosarcoidosis with optic neuropathies.

Tip: Sarcoidosis is a multisystem inflammatory disease characterized pathologically by chronic granulomatous inflammation of the lungs, skin and other internal organs. Up to 15 percent of patients with sarcoidosis have neurologic involvement known as Neurosarcoidosis, which may complicate systemic sarcoidosis, and sarcoidosis may present with isolated neurologic disease. Cranial neuropathies such as facial neuropathies and vestibulocochlear nerve impairment are common due to the predilection of the basilar meningeal involvement of neurosarcoidosis. This is an important mimicker of MS as it may cause optic neuropathies (as in this case) and spinal cord and cerebral parenchymal brain lesions.

Case 34: A 56-year-old man with fatigue, muscle pain and recurrent episodes of visual loss

Three decades earlier, this patient had recurring headaches and experienced visual loss in the right eye with central blurring spreading to involve the entire right visual field. Soon after, he had similar symptoms in the left eye. He was hospitalized locally and diagnosed with retrobulbar optic neuritis and treated with corticosteroids. He had complete bilateral blindness for one year. His vision gradually improved, but since that time he had repeated episodes of visual deficit in the right eye. These were each treated with oral corticosteroids. He had symptoms of generalized diffuse myalgias in the upper extremities. While he was formerly an avid runner, he now becomes fatigued easily and does not recover from running like he used to. A muscle biopsy was reported to be normal, as was his serum creatine kinase level.

The patient's older brother had a similar episode of visual loss in his thirties. A younger brother was unaffected. A maternal uncle became blind in his thirties. The patient's mother had a history of strokes but no visual deficits. The patient had two sons who were currently healthy and unaffected by visual impairment.

On neurological examination his mental status was found to be normal. He had bilateral visual acuity impairment and bilateral optic disc pallor with normal retinal background. Color vision was absent bilaterally. Motor power and reflexes were normal with flexor plantar responses. A sensory examination was normal.

A brain MRI scan showed a few punctate areas of nonspecific abnormal T2 signal consistent with small-vessel ischemic changes without change over five years. Genetic testing for Leber's hereditary optic neuropathy (LHON) was consistent with a pathological mutation.

Three-step assessment

1 Classical clinical features of MS: optic neuropathies
2 Neurological examination: bilateral severe optic neuropathies
3 Investigations: MRI brain not consistent with MS; genetic testing confirmatory of alternative disease of Leber's hereditary optic neuropathy (LHON)

Diagnosis: Leber's hereditary optic neuropathy (LHON).

Tip: Leber's hereditary optic neuropathy (LHON) is a mitochondrial disease. Individuals who carry mutant mitochondria, especially women, may not be clinically affected. One of the common mutations found in LHON at nucleotide position 14,484 was found in the patient's DNA. Genetic counseling is important for patients with LHON and their family members.

Further reading

McClelland CM, Van Stavern GP, Tselis AC. Leber hereditary optic neuropathy mimicking neuromyelitis optica. *J Neuroophthalmol* 2011;**31**:265–8.

Purvin V, Sundaram S, Neuroretinitis KA. Review of the literature and new observations. *J Neuroophthalmol* 2011;**31**:58–68.

Schrier SA, Falk MJ. Mitochondrial disorders and the eye. *Curr Opin Ophthalmol* 2011;**22**:325–31.

Friedman DI, Liu GT, Digre KB. Revised diagnostic criteria for the pseudotumor cerebri syndrome in adults and children. *Neurology* 2013;**81**:1159–65.

Pfeffer G, Burke A, Yu-Wai-Man P, Compston DA, Chinnery PF. Clinical features of MS associated with Leber hereditary optic neuropathy mtDNA mutations. *Neurology* 2013;**81**:2073–81.

Kosmorsky GS. Idiopathic intracranial hypertension: pseudotumor cerebri. *Headache* 2014;**54**:389–93.

Krumholz A, Stern BJ. Neurologic manifestations of sarcoidosis. *Handb Clin Neurol* 2014;**119**:305–33.

Qureshi SS, Beh SC, Frohman TC, Frohman EM. An update on neuro-ophthalmology of multiple sclerosis: the visual system as a model to study multiple sclerosis. *Curr Opin Neurol* 2014;**27**:300–8.

Du Y, Li JJ, Zhang YJ, Li K, He JF. Risk factors for idiopathic optic neuritis recurrence. *PLoS One* 2014;**9**:e108580.

Lim YM, Pyun SY, Lim HT, Jeong IH, Kim KK. First-ever optic neuritis: distinguishing subsequent neuromyelitis optica from multiple sclerosis. *Neurol Sci* 2014;**35**:781–3.

Pula JH, Kattah JC, Keung B, Wang H, Daily J. Longitudinally extensive optic neuritis in neuromyelitis optica spectrum disorder. *J Neurol Sci* 2014;**345**:209–12.

Pitfalls in diagnosing cerebral parenchymal disease

The majority of the CNS white matter lies within the cerebral hemispheres. Multiple sclerosis may present with a hemiparesis or hemisensory deficit when the white matter of the internal capsule is affected or if a particularly large MS lesion develops within the larger portion of the cerebral white matter. As most MS demyelinating lesions are of a relatively small size, many new inflammatory MS lesions of the cerebral white matter are clinically asymptomatic. When there are numerous MS lesions within the cerebral hemispheres, significant cognitive impairment may result. Demyelination within the cerebral cortex itself that is not easily apparent on a routine brain MRI is becoming more greatly appreciated. Seizures are slightly more common in MS than in the general population and may be due to involvement of the cortical white matter; however, seizures remain a relatively uncommon MS symptom. Many other disease processes may affect the cerebrum and potentially occur as MS mimickers.

Case 35: A 44-year-old gentleman with an 8-year history of cognitive impairment and possible MS

The patient's first neurological symptom arose eight years prior to presentation with a subacute onset of right upper extremity clumsiness. He recalled right arm weakness and gait ataxia accompanying this impairment, but the symptoms improved spontaneously. He had no other symptoms of optic neuritis or diplopia, nor other symptoms characteristic of MS attacks. Since that time, however, he has had progressive memory impairment. He became sloppy and inconsistent in his occupation as a farmer and could no longer balance his family and business finances. The patient was a long-term smoker and was unable to discontinue cigarette smoking. He had no family history of multiple sclerosis or any dementing disorders.

On neurological examination, he scored 21 out of 38 on the Kokmen short test of mental status (29/38 or less in this age group is consistent with dementia), revealing impairment through delayed recall and attention. A formal neuropsychological evaluation was compatible with a "subcortical" process affecting executive function, cognitive speed and flexibility. His motor examination was normal throughout, as were his reflexes. Plantar responses were extensor on the right and flexor on the left.

A repeat brain MRI showed areas of abnormal T2 signal, all of which were highly consistent with multiple sclerosis with only minimal change in signal abnormality over the next decade (Figure 6.1). A CSF examination showed elevated oligoclonal bands with normal CSF neuron-specific enolase (NSE) and 14–3–3 protein levels.

Three-step assessment

1 Classical clinical features of MS: hemiataxia with resolution, dementia
2 Neurological examination: dementia with corticospinal tract impairment (extensor plantar reflex)
3 Investigations: MRI brain consistent with MS; CSF consistent with MS

Diagnosis: Dementia due to multiple sclerosis.

Tip: Cognitive impairment due to multiple sclerosis can occur without significant motor or sensory impairment, even over many years. Cognitive impairment may be severe enough to warrant a diagnosis of significant dementia. Patients that smoke cigarettes appear to be overrepresented in the population of MS patients with significant dementia.

Case 36: A woman with MS and severe memory loss

A 53-year-old woman had transient true spinning vertigo lasting one week six years prior to evaluation.

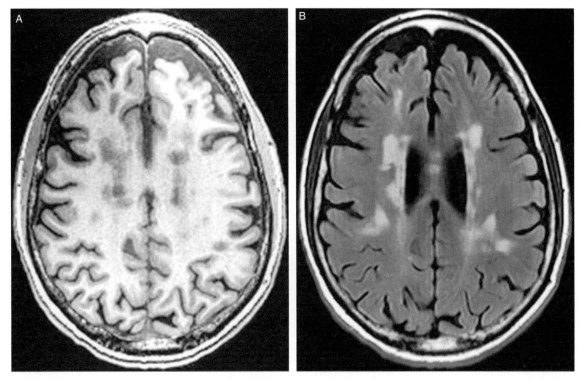

Figure 6.1 An axial T1 and FLAIR MRI brain scan shows numerous white matter lesions involving cerebral hemispheres ovoid in shape and periventricular in location, which is consistent with multiple sclerosis. Many white matter lesions demonstrated T1 hypointensity consistent with neuronal loss ("T1 black holes"). Mild generalized cerebral volume loss was noted. The pons and left middle cerebellar peduncle were also involved (not shown).

The following year she developed right upper extremity numbness and significant gait ataxia, again with resolution. Two years following that, she had insidiously progressive memory impairment. She was unable to manage her own finances for the prior four years, and she could not prepare meals any longer as she would forget the ingredients. She would leave tap water running and forget to turn it off. She could not reliably dress herself independently and she discontinued driving. She was poor at calculations, could not write, or focus her attention to play cards. She had a history of mood disorder with depression and anxiety, but this was stable and had not worsened.

On neurological examination, she scored 14 out of 38 on a Kokmen short test of mental status, displaying abnormalities on orientation, attention, registration, calculation and delayed recall. On language testing, she had impaired comprehension, mild difficulty with naming and moderate difficulty with repetition and writing. She had evidence of upper extremity ideomotor apraxia and palmar grasp response bilaterally with some pseudobulbar affect. A motor examination was normal but plantar responses were extensor bilaterally. Her walking revealed gait initiation failure (gait "apraxia").

Brain and spinal cord (not shown) MRI scans were highly consistent with multiple sclerosis (Figure 6.2 A). A CSF examination showed elevated oligoclonal bands and revealed tau and amyloid-b1–42 metabolites and amyloid-b1–42/tau index changes, reflecting a high sensitivity 85–94 percent and specificity 83–89 percent for Alzheimer's disease (Figure 6.2 B). A brain 18 F-fluorodeoxyglucose-PET (FDG-PET) revealed bilateral (left greater than right) fronto-temporal-parietal and posterior cingulate hypometabolism, highly suggestive of Alzheimer's disease (Figure 6.2 C).

Three-step assessment

1. Classical clinical features of MS: vertigo, ataxia, hemisensory symptoms with resolution, progressive severe dementia
2. Neurological examination: very severe dementia with corticospinal tract impairment

3 Investigations: MRI brain consistent with MS; CSF consistent with MS; CSF tau and amyloid-B1–42 metabolites consistent with Alzheimer's disease; PET brain consistent with Alzheimer's disease

Diagnosis: Multiple sclerosis with Alzheimer's disease.

Tip: Cortical symptoms and more severe signs of dementia may herald an alternative accompanying dementing disorder in addition to a history of multiple sclerosis. Novel new biomarkers for Alzheimer's disease including brain FDG-PET and CSF tau and Abeta metabolites can diagnose this condition in life. Occasional cases of MS complicated by Alzheimer's disease have been confirmed at autopsy. Confirmation of this unusual presentation may provide opportunities to treat Alzheimer's disease confidently with acetylcholinesterase inhibitors that have proven but modest benefits.

Case 37: A middle-aged man with progressive, treatment-resistant hemiparesis

A 52-year-old man presented with progressive left facial weakness, followed over the next few weeks and months by slowly progressive left upper and lower extremity weakness with dysarthria. He also had a significant personality change; specifically, he was previously felt to be very driven and ambitious and was now far more "easygoing." He had no other symptoms of MS attacks. There was no family history of MS. Intravenous corticosteroids were given without any improvement. He initiated treatment with interferon beta-1A intramuscular injections weekly along with monthly prednisolone infusions for a suspected diagnosis of MS. He started to use a cane initially and before long required a wheelchair.

On neurological examination he was inattentive and mildly inappropriate but was found to have no other impairment on mental status examination. He had no visuospatial neglect and his visual fields were full, and he had no papilledema. He had saccadic breakdown of smooth pursuit eye movements, and spastic dysarthria. A motor examination revealed left upper motor neuron-type facial weakness with severe spastic left hemiparesis. Right motor power was normal. Plantar responses were extensor on the left and flexor on the right. Cortical-type and other sensory exams were normal. He was wheelchair bound.

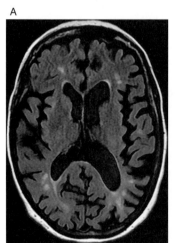

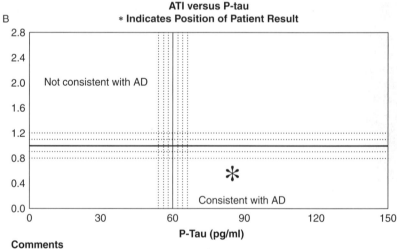

Comments

This analysis detected levels of $AB_{(1-42)}$ peptide, total tau and phospho-tau protein in cerebrospinal fluid which which are consistent with a diagnosis of Alzheimer's disease (AD) as a cause of his/her neurological symptoms.1-11

Figure 6.2 A) Axial T1 and FLAIR MRI brain scans showed periventricular and subcortical scattered T2 hyperintensities oriented perpendicularly to the lateral ventricles with moderate cerebral atrophy with bilateral frontoparietal predominance, slightly more pronounced on the left. A cervical spine MRI (not shown) demonstrated multiple discontinuous foci of T2 hyperintensity from the C2 level to C5 involving the posterior and/or lateral aspects of the spinal cord. B) CSF revealed tau and amyloid-b1–42 metabolites and amyloid-b1–42/tau index changes reflecting a high probability of Alzheimer's disease. C) Brain 18 F-fluorodeoxyglucose-PET (FDG-PET) showed bilateral (left greater than right) fronto-temporal-parietal and posterior cingulate hypometabolism, highly suggestive of Alzheimer's disease.

C

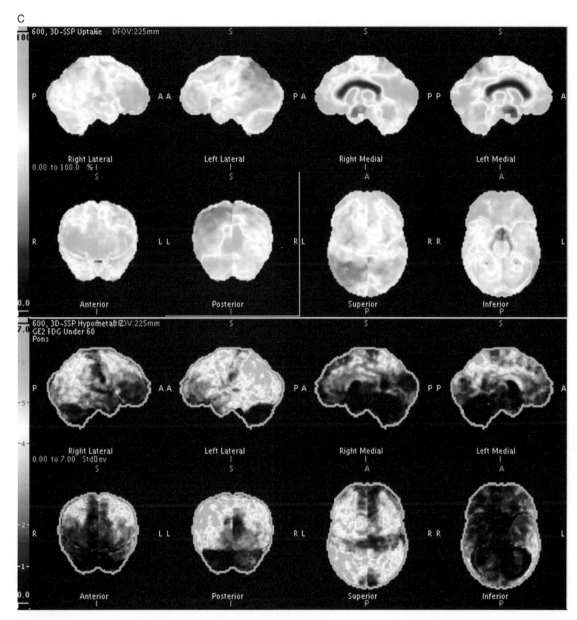

Figure 6.2 (cont.)

A brain MRI showed greater T2 signal abnormality in the right than left hemisphere white matter with an area of abnormal T2 signal within the pons (Figure 6.3). There was evidence of mass effect as well as subtle gadolinium enhancement. Cervical and thoracic spinal cord MRIs were normal. A CSF examination was normal without oligoclonal bands or elevations in IgG index and a cytology was negative for malignancy. A CSF was negative for Lyme disease, Whipple's agent, syphilis, angiotensin converting enzyme (ACE), tuberculosis, West Nile virus, herpes simplex virus and John Cunningham (JC) virus polymerase chain reaction (PCR). Fungi and bacterial cultures were all negative. A brain biopsy confirmed pathological evidence of gliomatosis cerebri.

Three-step assessment

1 Classical clinical features of MS: progressive hemiparesis, but treatment-resistant with personality change

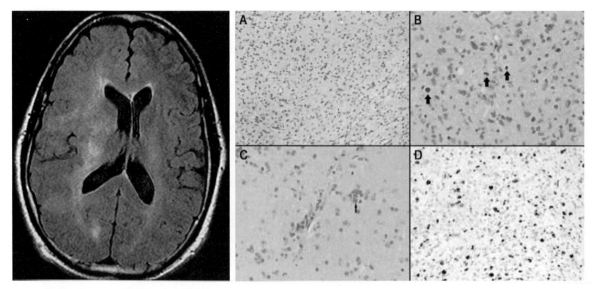

Figure 6.3 A) Axial FLAIR MRI shows a bilateral, asymmetric diffuse white matter process that extends from the pons through the midbrain (not shown) into the deep white matter of both cerebral hemispheres. There is mass effect with effacement of several sulci and shift of midline structures to the left. The imaging findings are most consistent with a diffusely infiltrative process such as a glioma. B) Hematoxylin eosin stains show elongated, pleomorphic neoplastic cells diffusely infiltrating cerebral parenchyma with evidence of perineuronal satellites, perivascular neoplastic aggregates and numerous mitotic figures.

2   Neurological examination: upper motor neuron hemiparesis with inattention and mildly inappropriate behavior

3   Investigations: MRI brain not consistent with MS; MRI spinal cord not consistent with MS; CSF not consistent with MS; brain biopsy confirmatory of primary brain neoplasm

   Diagnosis: Gliomatosis cerebri.

   Tip: The patient progressed to death 14 months later. The progressive nature of the patient's worsening that was treatment-resistant along with atypical MRI features, a normal CSF and a normal MRI scan of the spine indicated an alternative diagnosis to that of multiple sclerosis. Gliomatosis cerebri is a diffusely infiltrating astrocytoma that affects multiple lobes. Mass effect and gadolinium enhancement may not be seen, particularly early in the clinical course. Median survival has been estimated at between 6 and 39 months.

Case 38: A man with progressive white matter disease and an "alien" limb

A 41-year-old man presented with progressive left upper and lower stiffness. He exhibited left upper extremity limb apraxia and "alien limb" phenomenon, which manifested as his hand involuntarily grabbing onto his shirt repetitively. He developed bilateral lower extremity weakness as well as a spastic dysarthria. He had no family history of any neurological diseases including MS or leukoencephalopathy. Serological testing was negative for inherited, acquired and other degenerative leukoencephalopathies known at the time.

On neurological examination he had mild impairment on a Kokmen short test of mental status, scoring 34/38 and missing elements on orientation, construction and delayed recall. Cranial nerves were normal, including color vision. He had an upper motor neuron spastic dysarthria, with a brisk jaw jerk. He had a moderate left greater than right hemiparesis, with normal sensation walking with a left hemiparetic gait. He had a grasp reflex and apraxia of the left upper extremity.

Serial brain MRIs showed progressive, asymmetrical confluent white matter abnormalities without gadolinium enhancement (Figure 6.4 A). Cervical and thoracic spinal cord MRI scans were normal. A CSF examination was normal apart from a moderate increase in neuron-specific enolase (NSE) without elevations in either oligoclonal bands or IgG index. A brain biopsy showed axonal spheroids appearing as

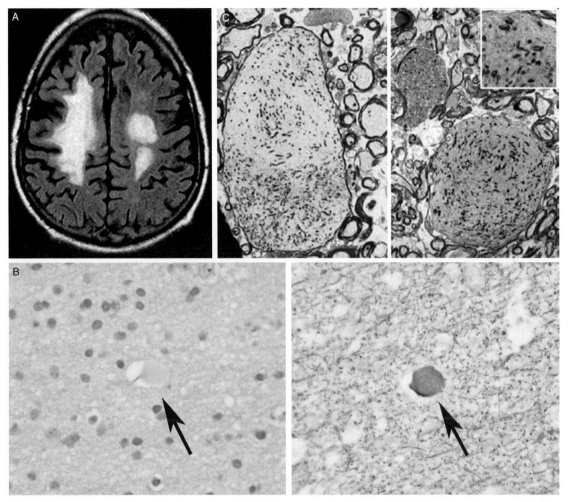

Figure 6.4 A) Axial FLAIR MRI brain showing moderate to marked confluent non-enhancing T2 foci in the right greater than left cerebral hemispheric white matter (from BM Keegan *et al.*, 2008 with permission). B) Brain biopsy showing axonal spheroids appearing as pale eosinophilic globules on hematoxylin and eosin staining. C) Electron microscopy of the brain pathology demonstrated axonal spheroids within the white matter (from BM Keegan et al., 2008, with permission).

pale eosinophilic globules on hematoxylin and eosin staining (Figure 6.4 B). An electron microscopy of the brain pathology demonstrated axonal spheroids within the white matter (Figure 6.4 C).

Three-step assessment

1 Classical clinical features of MS: progressive upper motor neuron quadriparesis
2 Neurological examination: asymmetric upper motor neuron quadriparesis with alien limb phenomenon and signs of frontal lobe dysfunction
3 Investigations: MRI brain not consistent with MS; MRI spinal cord not consistent with MS; CSF not consistent with MS; brain biopsy confirmatory of sporadic adult onset

leukoencephalopathy with neuroaxonal spheroids

Diagnosis: Sporadic adult-onset leukoencephalopathy with neuroaxonal spheroids mimicking multiple sclerosis.

Tip: Important considerations in this case are the progressive nature of the impairment, confluent white matter abnormalities associated with significant atrophy, the lack of gadolinium-enhancing lesions or focal lesions and the lack of spinal cord MRI findings as well as a lack of abnormalities on CSF examination. Brain MRIs may show focal areas of restricted diffusion, particularly in patients with rapid onset of sporadic adult-onset leukoencephalopathy with neuroaxonal spheroids. Familial cases of neuroaxonal

55

spheroids with leukoencephalopathy have been described as well. The genetic mutation has been found to be in the colony-stimulating factor 1 receptor (CSF1R) gene, causing hereditary diffuse leukoencephalopathy with spheroids. Whether this genetic mutation is responsible for sporadic cases currently remains uncertain.

Case 39: A man with an abnormal brain MRI and a persistently enhancing cervical spine MRI lesion for possible MS

A 46-year-old gentleman recalled awakening one morning with right arm weakness and numbness. Within about three days, however, the symptoms resolved and these areas returned to normal power and sensation. He would sometimes "lose his train of thought" but had no major cognitive impairment. He had no prior symptoms of optic neuritis, diplopia, dysarthria or dysphagia. He did not have a Lhermitte symptom nor bowel or bladder incontinence, but suffered from urinary hesitancy and incomplete bladder emptying which was attributed to benign prostatic hyperplasia. He had no reported family history of multiple sclerosis, dementia or

any other neurological disease. A possible diagnosis of multiple sclerosis was raised and he initiated interferon beta 1-a intramuscular injections once weekly but had to discontinue after getting flu-like symptoms and fever one to three days following the injections.

On neurological examination, he scored 35/38 on a Kokmen short test of mental status. His visual fields were full. Pupils were symmetrical and normal. Extraocular movements were full and normal. Speech was clear. A motor exam was found to be normal and his reflexes were brisk, but his plantar responses were flexor bilaterally. In addition, a sensory exam and his gait and coordination were normal.

A brain MRI showed multiple areas of abnormal T2 signal throughout without enhancement, including signal abnormality in the tips of the temporal lobes bilaterally (Figure 6.5). A cervical spine MRI showed an enhancing lesion at C3-C4 within the cord (Figure 6.6). Repeated cervical spine MRIs continued to show the same enhancing intramedullary lesion at the C3-C4 level that was unchanged in appearance with no associated blood products. An incidental occult vascular malformation such as capillary telangiectasia was therefore suspected. A CSF examination was normal without elevations in oligoclonal bands or IgG index. Visual evoked

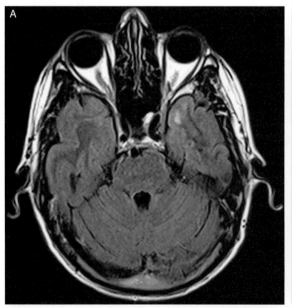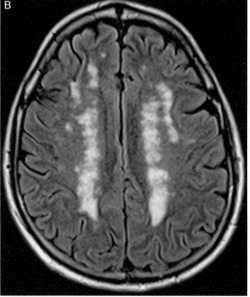

Figure 6.5 Axial FLAIR MRI shows T2 signal abnormality in the tip of the anterior left temporal lobe. Multiple non-enhancing periventricular and subcortical T2 lesions are seen throughout both cerebral hemispheres.

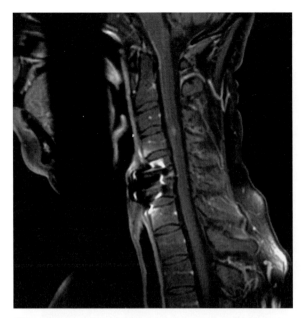

Figure 6.6 Sagittal T1 with gadolinium cervical spine MRI shows an entirely stable and persistently and chronically enhancing intramedullary lesion at C3-C4 consistent with a capillary telangiectasia. There was prior anterior cervical fusion at the C5-C6 level with no other intramedullary lesions identified throughout the spinal cord.

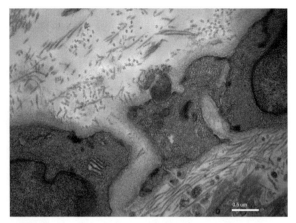

Figure 6.7 Skin biopsy electron microscopy showing disorganization of the walls of the vascular smooth muscle cells, thickened basal lamina and deposits of granular osmiophilic material (GOM) characteristic of CADASIL.

potentials were normal. A skin biopsy studied by electron microscopy was performed (Figure 6.7). Special attention to dermal vessels demonstrated disorganization of the walls of the vascular smooth muscle cells. The basal lamina was thickened and distorted by irregular deposits of granular osmiophilic material (GOM), all of which features were characteristic of CADASIL (cerebral autosomal dominant arteriopathy with subcortical infarcts and leukoencephalopathy). Genetic testing confirmed a DNA sequence alteration and in the NOTCH3 gene diagnostic of CADASIL.

Three-step assessment
1. Classical clinical features of MS: transient arm weakness and numbness
2. Neurological examination: normal
3. Investigations: MRI brain not consistent with MS; CSF not consistent with MS; visual evoked potentials normal; skin biopsy and genetic testing diagnostic of CADASIL

   Diagnosis: Cerebral autosomal dominant arteriopathy with subcortical infarcts and leukoencephalopathy (CADASIL).

Tip: Extension of T2 signal into the tips of the temporal lobes is consistent with brain MRI features of CADASIL. Persistently enhancing spinal cord lesion without change over time suggests a vascular malformation such as a capillary telangiectasia rather than an acute demyelinating lesion of MS where gadolinium enhancement resolves within 8–12 weeks in most cases.

Case 40: A woman with breast cancer, obstructive hydrocephalus and corpus callosum abnormalities

A 55-year-old woman was referred for a second opinion as to whether MRI lesions associated with obstructive hydrocephalus were demyelinating in nature.

The woman had known metastatic breast cancer to the spinal vertebral bodies with prior chemotherapy and focal spinal irradiation. She developed a holocephalic headache associated with vomiting and was found to have obstructive hydrocephalus. She was treated with dexamethasone and ultimately a ventriculoperitoneal shunt was placed, and after adjustment of the pressure she had relief of her headaches. She had no limb coordination symptoms, diplopia or any other neurological symptoms. There were not remote symptoms suggestive of MS attacks with resolution and no family history of multiple sclerosis.

On neurologic examination, her mental status was normal, she had no papilledema and extraocular movements and pupil responses were normal.

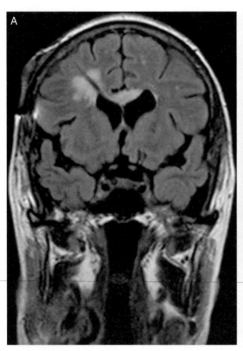
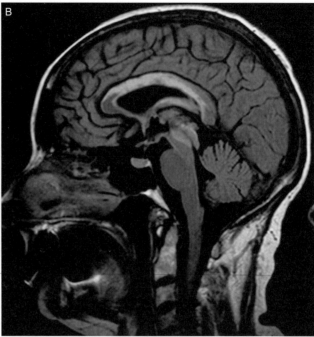

Figure 6.8 Coronal and sagittal FLAIR MRI brain showing a non-enhancing mass within the midbrain tectum with prominent T2 signal within the corpus callosum related to a corpus callosal crush injury from hydrocephalus; a ventricular shunt tube has been placed through a right frontal burr hole to relieve acute obstructive hydrocephalus.

A motor examination, reflexes and gait were all normal. Plantar responses were flexor bilaterally. A brain MRI showed obstructive hydrocephalus due to a midbrain lesion with dilatation of the lateral and third ventricles with improvement following shunt placement (Figure 6.8). There was increased T2/FLAIR signal greater on the left than the right surrounding the cerebral aqueduct and T2 signal of the corpus callosum following shunting likely due to a corpus callosal crush injury from the hydrocephalus. A CSF cytology was negative, there were no oligoclonal bands and the IgG index was normal.

Three-step assessment

1. Classical clinical features of MS: None
2. Neurological examination: normal
3. Investigations: MRI brain not consistent with MS, consistent with corpus callosum changes due to ventriculoperitoneal shunting; CSF not consistent with MS

   Diagnosis: Metastatic breast cancer with corpus callosal signal changes due to ventriculoperitoneal shunting for obstructive hydrocephalus.

   Tip: Demyelinating lesions due to MS would not be expected to cause any CSF disruption and

subsequent obstructive hydrocephalus. Diffuse corpus callosum abnormalities related to shunted hydrocephalus have been reported and should not be confused for another inflammatory, infiltrative or demyelinating white matter disease in this clinical context.

Case 41: A woman with subacute psychiatric symptoms, mutism and involuntary orofacial and limb movements

A 27-year-old woman was well until she had complaints of insomnia. She then developed psychiatric symptoms with generalized anxiety and severe emotional lability which were highly atypical for her. She became fixated on the idea that she was pregnant despite repeated negative home pregnancy tests. She then developed pressured speech and progressively worsening confusion, anxiety and insomnia. She was admitted to a psychiatric unit with agitation and combativeness requiring antipsychotic medications. Her blood pressure was labile; she became tachycardic and had body

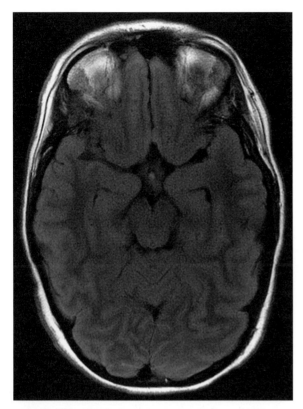

Figure 6.9 Axial FLAIR MRI brain normal with no mass lesion, no abnormal T2 FLAIR hyperintensity within the temporal lobes, including the hippocampi.

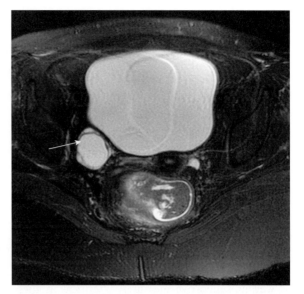

Figure 6.10 MRI pelvis showing a 3.2 cm benign-appearing cystic lesion in the right ovary with tiny focus of mural fat, suggestive of small ovarian teratoma.

temperatures up to 100.4° Fahrenheit, requiring transfer to the medical intensive care unit. Urinalysis and evaluation for drugs of abuse were negative. She had worsening distractibility, flight of ideas, increased activity, agitation and insomnia. She then developed abnormal, repetitive orofacial dyskinesias and involuntary upper limb movements.

On neurological examination she was inattentive and mute and did not follow commands. She had numerous orofacial movements and involuntary twitching. There was no motor impairment and her plantar responses were bilaterally flexor.

A brain MRI showed no significant abnormalities (Figure 6.9). A CSF examination showed a white blood cell count of 43 with 93 percent lymphocytes. The CSF showed protein and glucose levels were normal and herpes simplex virus polymerase chain reaction (PCR) was negative. Her CSF IgG index was normal at 0.65 but seven unique CSF oligoclonal bands were found. CSF antibodies to the N-methyl-

D-aspartate receptor (NMDA-R) by cell-binding assay were positive, consistent with NMDA-associated encephalitis. An EEG initially showed diffuse slowing most prominent over the right temporal region and then frequent, independent, bitemporal focal seizures without clinical correlate.

An abdomen and pelvis computed tomography (CT) showed no malignancy. A pelvic ultrasound showed a 2.3 cm × 1.5 cm × 2.6 cm right ovarian mass consistent with a corpus luteal cyst. A pelvis MRI showed a benign-appearing cystic lesion in the right ovary with tiny focus of mural fat suggestive of a small ovarian teratoma (Figure 6.10). A fallopian tube and right ovarian salpingo-oophorectomy was performed, where a mature ovarian teratoma was excised. A predominant component of skin and adnexa, mature respiratory epithelium and focal mature neural elements were found in the tumor.

She was treated with corticosteroids, intravenous immunoglobulin (IVIG) and rituximab. She was on antiepileptic medications, which controlled seizures. Slow but steady improvement was noted over many months.

Three-step assessment

1 Classical clinical features of MS: not typical of MS; subacute encephalopathy with prominent psychiatric symptoms, orofacial and limb dyskinesias

2 Neurological examination: consistent with alternative diagnosis orofacial dyskinesias, mutism

3 Investigations: MRI brain not consistent with MS; MRI spinal cord not consistent with MS; CSF oligoclonal bands, with NMDA receptor antibodies; ovarian biopsy confirmatory of ovarian teratoma

Diagnosis: NMDA receptor antibody encephalitis with ovarian teratoma.

Tip: The onset of psychiatric symptoms – the orofacial and upper extremity twitching and dyskinesias followed by significant autonomic dysfunction and catatonia – are hallmark features of NMDA receptor-associated encephalitis. An ovarian teratoma is commonly found, as in this case. A high suspicion is required to investigate this type of teratoma and initial evaluations were unrevealing in this patient. Excision of the tumor and intensive immunotherapy, as well as supportive measures, is critical in these patients. Improvement often takes many months and relapses may occur.

Case 42: A young woman with repetitive brief episodes of hemiparesis and dysarthria and progressive brain MRI abnormalities

A 32-year-old woman was brought to medical attention three years previously for alcohol abuse. She presented with right upper extremity numbness and incoordination lasting ten minutes. Three months later, she developed left face, arm, and leg paralysis with dysarthria initially lasting 30 minutes with subsequent repetitive episodes of left-sided paresis and dysarthria, each of 10–15 minutes' duration.

Eighteen months later, she fell while walking and was very confused for two weeks. She then had a significant personality change, altering from previously being very headstrong and now becoming much easier to get along with. Her mother described her as though acting "like a child."

The patient had a long history of alcohol abuse but had been sober for the last three years. She had smoked between one and two packs of cigarettes per day continuously since she was age 14. She admitted to intranasal and smoking cocaine and heroin, as well as the oral use of ephedrine. She denied having a history of methamphetamine or any injectable illicit drug use in the past. She was considered to

possibly have multiple sclerosis on the basis of the progressive abnormal signal on brain MRI scans.

On neurological examination, she scored normally on a short test of mental status but was distractible and behaviorally inappropriate at times. Her neurological examination otherwise was normal.

A brain MRI showed significant T2 abnormality in both cerebral white matter associated with T1 hypointensity in the left hemispheric white matter (Figure 6.11). There was gadolinium enhancement involving the right hemispheric white matter which had progressed from prior brain MRIs. A cervical spine MRI was normal. A CSF examination was normal, with no oligoclonal bands or elevation in IgG index. An EEG showed right frontal slowing without seizures. An extensive battery for connective tissue disease and inherited leukodystrophies was negative. An MR angiography showed evidence of severe stenosis involving the distal carotids, proximal middle cerebral artery and anterior cerebral artery territories consistent with prior arteritis and Moyamoya syndrome (Figure 6.11).

Three-step assessment

1 Classical clinical features of MS: brief episodes of hemisensory deficit, dysarthria, more consistent with transient ischemic attacks, progressive cognitive disorder

2 Neurological examination: cognitive disorder with suggestion of frontal lobe dysfunction

3 Investigations: MRI brain not consistent with MS; MRI cervical spinal cord not consistent with MS; CSF examination normal; MRA and cerebral angiography confirmed moyamoya

Diagnosis: Moyamoya syndrome due to sympathicomimetic drug associated vasculitis.

Tip: Her clinical history with sudden onset of repetitive symptoms suggests a vascular rather than a demyelinating cause, which would typically progress over hours and be maintained for days to weeks. An initial evaluation of the angiography results indicated they were normal. A thorough imaging review later demonstrated the abnormalities. Her presentation was likely secondary to sympathomimetic drug vasculitis. A bilateral superficial temporal to middle cerebral artery (STA-MCA) bypass was performed to allow blood flow to bypass proximal lesions of the intracranial vasculature and to encourage subsequent neovascularization.

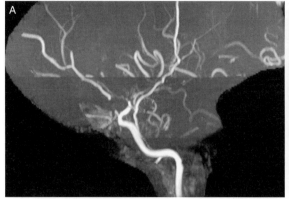
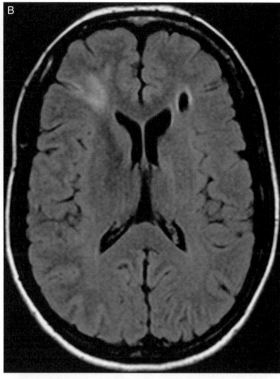

Figure 6.11 A) Intracranial MR angiography demonstrates stenotic changes in both intracranial carotid systems most notable at the carotid terminus bilaterally with areas of stenosis within the distal internal carotid arteries and proximal middle and anterior cerebral arteries. The findings are consistent with changes due to arteritis and the anatomic locations of the abnormalities are consistent with Moyamoya disease. B) Axial FLAIR MRI demonstrates multiple areas of infarction involving the deep white matter of the frontal lobes bilaterally with cavitation on the left.

Case 43: A man with bladder incontinence, progressive gait impairment and brain white matter lesions

A 63-year-old gentleman presented with a one-and-a-half year history of progressive walking impairment with his right leg being worse than the left. He had symptoms of neurogenic bladder dysfunction with bladder incontinence for one decade prior to presentation. He had no impairment of memory or problems with his vision, hearing or upper extremities.

His family history revealed that his father had progressive gait disorder and now walked with two canes, and a brother had progressive gait impairment with leg weakness which required use of a walker. A sister had been diagnosed with possible multiple sclerosis. The patient himself had three children, none of whom had walking difficulties.

On neurological examination, his mental status was found to be normal and he had normal motor power throughout and sensory examination was normal. Reflexes were normal, but plantar responses were extensor bilaterally.

A brain MRI showed evidence of confluent, non-enhancing white matter T2 hyperintensity in the subcortical region with abnormal signal in the corticospinal tracts, middle cerebellar peduncles, the dorsal midbrain, and medulla (Figure 6.12). A spinal cord MRI showed lateral corticospinal T2 signal abnormalities with symmetric spinal cord atrophy (Figure 6.13). Genetic testing was negative for the DARS2 mutation in aspartyl-tRNA-synthetase. Genetic testing was positive for the duplication of the Lamin B1 (LMNB1) gene consistent with a diagnosis of autosomal-dominant leukodystrophy.

Three-step assessment

1 Classical clinical features of MS: progressive myelopathy

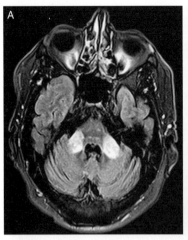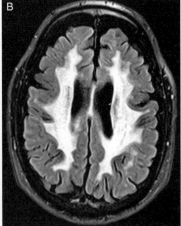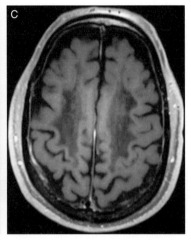

Figure 6.12 Axial FLAIR and T1 MRI brain shows extensive confluent non-enhancing white matter T2 hyperintensity, with T1 hypointensity involving the cerebral hemispheres, most marked periventricularly involving the dorsal midbrain, and cerebellar peduncles, with marked involvement of the middle cerebral peduncles and the medulla without enhancement. Generalized cerebral and cerebellar volume loss is demonstrated.

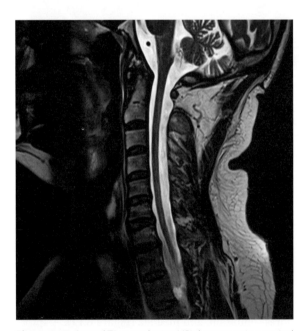

Figure 6.13 Sagittal T2 cervical spine MRI shows prominent spinal cord atrophy.

2 Neurological examination: consistent with myelopathy
3 Investigations: MRI brain not consistent with MS; MRI spinal cord not consistent with MS; genetic testing duplication of the Lamin B1 (LMNB1) gene diagnostic of autosomal-dominant leukodystrophy

Diagnosis: Autosomal-dominant leukodystrophy due to the duplication of the Lamin B1 (LMNB1) gene.

Tip: Early onset of autonomic symptoms such as bladder impairment and orthostatic lightheadedness can be prominent with autosomal-dominant leukodystrophy. Memory is commonly preserved early on, as it was in this case, but progressive gait impairment with imbalance, spasticity and leg weakness occurs. Lamins are components of the nuclear lamina, a fibrous layer on the nucleoplasmic side of the inner nuclear membrane. The autosomal-dominated inheritance means a risk factor of 50 percent for each child of an infected individual to inherit the Lamin B1 duplication. Pathologically oligodendroglia cells are preserved despite demyelination.

Further reading

Staff NP, Lucchinetti CF, Keegan BM. Multiple sclerosis with predominant, severe cognitive impairment. *Arch Neurol* 2009;**66**:1139–43.

Kokmen E, Naessens J, Offord K. A short test of mental status: Description and preliminary results. *Mayo Clin Proc* 1987;**62**:281–8.

Zarei M, Chandran S, Compston A, Hodges J. Cognitive presentation of multiple sclerosis: evidence for a cortical variant. *Journal of Neurology, Neurosurgery & Psychiatry* 2003;**74**:872–7.

Rao SM, Leo GJ, Bernardin L, Unverzagt F. Cognitive dysfunction in multiple sclerosis. *I. Frequency, patterns, and prediction. Neurology* 1991;**41**:685–91.

Keegan BM, Giannini C, Parisi JE, Lucchinetti CF, Boeve BF, Josephs KA. Sporadic adult-onset leukoencephalopathy with neuroaxonal spheroids mimicking cerebral MS. *Neurology* 2008;**70**:1128–33.

Mateen FJ, Keegan BM, Krecke K, Parisi JE, Trenerry MR, Pittock SJ. Sporadic leucodystrophy with neuroaxonal spheroids: persistence of DWI changes and neurocognitive profiles: a case study. *Journal of neurology, neurosurgery, and psychiatry* 2010;**81**:619–22.

Fleming JO, Keegan BM, Parisi JE. A 52-year-old man with progressive left-sided weakness and white matter disease. *Neurology* 2007;**69**:600–6.

Padiath QS, Fu YH. Autosomal dominant leukodystrophy caused by lamin B1 duplications a clinical and molecular case study of altered nuclear function and disease. *Methods Cell Biol* 2010;**98**:337–57.

Dalmau J, Lancaster E, Martinez-Hernandez E, Rosenfeld MR, Balice-Gordon R. Clinical experience and laboratory investigations in patients with anti-NMDAR encephalitis. *Lancet Neurol* 2011;**10**:63–74.

Lin ST, Ptacek LJ, Fu YH. Adult-onset autosomal dominant leukodystrophy: linking nuclear envelope to myelin. *J Neurosci* 2011;**31**:1163–6.

Rademakers R, Baker M, Nicholson AM, et al. Mutations in the colony stimulating factor 1 receptor (CSF1 R) gene cause hereditary diffuse leukoencephalopathy with spheroids. *Nat Genet* 2012;**44**:200–5.

Jones KC, Benseler SM, Moharir M. Anti-NMDA Receptor Encephalitis. *Neuroimaging Clin N Am* 2013;**23**:309–20.

Nicholson AM, Baker MC, Finch NA, et al. CSF1 R mutations link POLD and HDLS as a single disease entity. *Neurology* 2013;**80**:1033–40.

Kronenburg A, Braun KP, van der Zwan A, Klijn CJ. Recent advances in moyamoya disease: pathophysiology and treatment. *Curr Neurol Neurosci Rep* 2014;**14**:423.

Chabriat H, Joutel A, Dichgans M, Tournier-Lasserve E, Bousser MG. Cadasil. *Lancet Neurol* 2009;**8**:643–53.

Constantinescu CS, McConachie NS, White BD. Corpus callosum changes following shunting for hydrocephalus: case report and review of the literature. *Clin Neurol Neurosurg* 2005;**107**:351–4.

Lane JI, Luetmer PH, Atkinson JL. Corpus callosal signal changes in patients with obstructive hydrocephalus after ventriculoperitoneal shunting. *AJNR Am J Neuroradiol* 2001;**22**:158–62.

Chapter 7

Pitfalls in diagnosing demyelinating cerebellar disease

The cerebellar outflow tracts and their connections to the brainstem are large white matter areas that are commonly affected by MS. Cerebellar impairment due to MS may occur both acutely due to new inflammatory MS lesions, as well as in a progressive fashion causing slowly progressive cerebellar ataxic presentations. Long-term MS–related ataxia is notoriously difficult to treat symptomatically. A number of neoplastic, inflammatory and degenerative diseases mimic cerebellar impairment due to MS and need to be confidently excluded when diagnosing MS.

Case 44: A middle-aged woman with a progressive right- then left-sided tremor

A 55-year-old woman presented with progressive impairment, suffering from tremors and incoordination of the right side that was greater than on the left. The right-sided symptoms had been progressive over the prior ten years and the left hand over the last three years prior to presentation. About 16 years prior to presentation she had painless, left-sided monocular visual loss with resolution. She was diagnosed with multiple sclerosis 14 years ago when she developed subacute dysarthria and right-sided incoordination and weakness which resolved itself. She initiated treatment with interferon beta 1-b subcutaneous every other day at that time.

She had a 45-pack-per-year history of cigarette smoking which she successfully discontinued six years ago. A maternal first cousin had multiple sclerosis. She can walk a couple of miles without difficulty despite the tremor. She had no further symptoms of new clinical attacks of multiple sclerosis with resolution.

On neurological examination her mental status and extraocular movements were normal, displaying no signs of internuclear ophthalmoplegia. She had a mild cerebellar dysarthric speech and mild head tremor with titubation. Her motor strength and reflexes were normal with bilateral flexor plantar responses. She had a moderate to severe postural and action tremor on the right upper extremity with a mild postural and action tremor on the left upper extremity. Her lower extremities suffered from no significant incoordination. Tandem walking was ataxic, but straight walking was only mildly impaired.

Brain MRI showed stable MS with posterior fossa and periventricular foci of non-enhancing T2 signal, some with T1 hypointensity consistent with chronic demyelinating plaques and mild to moderate diffuse cerebral atrophy (Figure 7.1).

Three-step assessment

1   Classical clinical features of MS: optic neuritis, progressive hemiataxia (bilateral)
2   Neurological examination: asymmetrical limb ataxia (cerebellar outflow tremor)
3   Investigations: MRI brain consistent with MS

   Diagnosis: Secondary Progressive MS with progressive cerebellar impairment.

   Tip: A cerebellar outflow tremor due to MS is notoriously difficult to treat symptomatically but benzodiazepines and gabapentin are often recommended.

Case 45: A woman with progressive cerebellar ataxia and an isolated cerebellar lesion. Is it MS?

A 71-year-old woman was well until two years prior to presentation. At that time, she had a relatively acute onset of vertigo and gait impairment. She continued to have worsening symptoms following the onset with progressive gait impairment. A brain MRI identified an enhancing lesion in the cerebellar hemisphere. She initiated treatments on corticosteroids, and a cerebellar biopsy was subsequently performed that was pathologically non-diagnostic, with evidence of gliosis but no neoplasm.

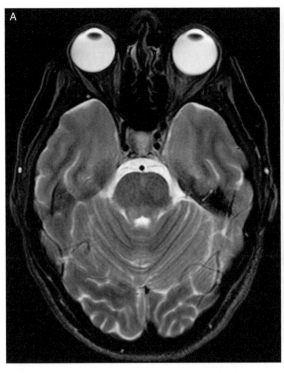
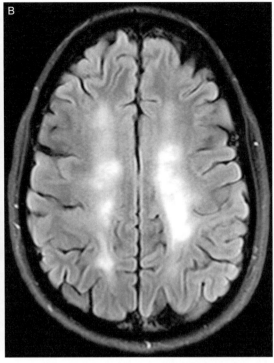

Figure 7.1 Axial T2 MRI brain showing abnormal focal T2 signal abnormalities within the pons and cerebellar peduncles and axial FLAIR MRI showing extensive, non-enhancing increased T2 signal in the periventricular white matter directly abutting the ventricles.

Since that time, she suffered from worsening incoordination of the right upper extremity. She had developed intractable hiccups, occasional diplopia and progressive truncal ataxia with worsening gait impairment. She initially started to use a walker but now required a wheelchair for ambulation. She had tapered off the corticosteroids entirely and had a brief course of cerebellar irradiation despite the lack of clear diagnosis. She had a 33-pack-per-year history of cigarette smoking. There was no family history of MS or other autoimmune CNS diseases.

On neurological examination she was awake and alert. She was severely debilitated, however, by the truncal ataxia. She had gaze-evoked horizontal nystagmus with macro square-wave jerks but no downbeat nystagmus. There was no palatal myoclonus. Motor examination was normal apart from being deconditioned. Plantar responses were flexor bilaterally. She had a tremor in the right greater side than on the left, with incoordination of both the upper and lower extremities and severe truncal ataxia which meant she found it difficult to even sit upright.

A repeat brain MRI showed a continuing area of abnormal T2 signal with gadolinium enhancement

(Figure 7.2). A CSF examination was found to be normal. CT scans of the chest, abdomen and pelvis were also normal. Repeat cerebellar biopsies demonstrated a low-grade astrocytoma with features consistent of a pilocytic astrocytoma (WHO grade I).

Three-step assessment

1 Classical clinical features of MS: progressive cerebellar ataxia
2 Neurological examination: consistent with cerebellar disease
3 Investigations: MRI brain not consistent with MS; MRI spinal cord not consistent with MS; repeat biopsy diagnostic of low-grade astrocytoma, pilocytic astrocytoma

Diagnosis: Cerebellar pilocytic astrocytoma (WHO grade I).

Tip: The patient had impairment restricted to the cerebellum only that was progressive over time. Despite the initial biopsy being unremarkable, she continued to worsen with severe gait impairment. A repeat brain biopsy may be needed in patients where the initial biopsy was felt to be non-diagnostic and there is continued progressive worsening.

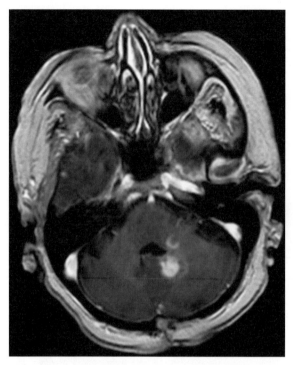

Figure 7.2 Axial T1 with gadolinium, an MRI brain showing an abnormal enhancing lesion within the left cerebellar hemisphere centered on the dentate nucleus and extending into the left middle cerebellar peduncle and left side of the brainstem.

Case 46: A young gentleman with acute onset of severe ataxia

A 27-year-old gentleman reported very brief episodes of true spinning vertigo lasting five to ten seconds in duration and which occurred while he was standing. He had no nausea, vomiting, tinnitus, dysarthria or dysphagia. He would have one episode per day and never more than that for the initial two weeks. He then awoke one morning with worsened and more persistent vertigo and painless, binocular, vertical diplopia. He then had progressive gait ataxia and dysarthria over three days. He was hospitalized and treated with intravenous corticosteroids for five days with initial symptomatic improvement. He then continued to deteriorate with more significant gait ataxia, dysarthria and diplopia. He had no cognitive impairment, visual loss, motor weakness, sensory loss or Lhermitte symptoms, or bowel or bladder dysfunction.

He had no prior neurological symptoms, no skin rash and no recent contact with anyone ill. He had no insect or tick bites and no farm animals or toxin exposures. There was no family history of neurological disease.

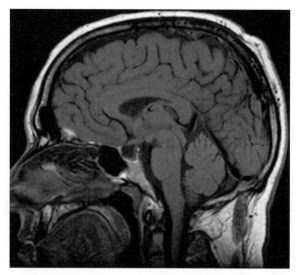

Figure 7.3 Sagittal T1 MRI head demonstrates subtle associated elevation of T1 signal on pre-contrast images with no definite contrast enhancement, mass-effect or atrophy. Subtle, but definite, high T2 signal involving the folia of both cerebellar hemispheres, left greater than right, was seen on FLAIR imaging (not shown). Diagnostic considerations include paraneoplastic syndromes and infectious and post-infectious cerebellitis.

A brain MRI showed a subtle increased T2 signal in the folia of both cerebellar hemispheres without contrast enhancement, mass effect or atrophy (Figure 7.3). A CSF examination showed 28 white blood cells with 83 percent lymphocytes, a protein of 40 mg/dL with negative oligoclonal bands and normal IgG index. Visual evoked potentials were normal. Infectious agents and a serum paraneoplastic antibody screen were negative. Chest, abdomen and pelvic CTs and a scrotal ultrasound were negative for neoplasms. A cerebellar biopsy showed findings consistent with acute cerebellar degeneration with marked Purkinje cell loss associated with Bergmann gliosis, white matter and molecular cell layer gliosis with scattered reactive T-lymphocytes. Microglial activation was observed without microglial nodules.

A follow-up brain MRI one year later showed interval progression of cerebellar atrophy without abnormal gadolinium enhancement and no other abnormalities.

Three-step assessment
1 Classical clinical features of MS: cerebellar ataxia, binocular painless diplopia
2 Neurological examination: severe, isolated cerebellar ataxia
3 Investigations: MRI brain not consistent with MS; CSF not consistent with MS; visual evoked

potentials normal; cerebellar biopsy, confirmatory of cerebellitis with cerebellar degeneration

Diagnosis: Acquired, presumably autoimmune, acute cerebellitis with subsequent cerebellar degeneration.

Tip: The acute and severe impairment in this patient with completely isolated involvement of the cerebellum is inconsistent with MS and consistent with cerebellitis. The brain MRI findings did not show typical white matter disease characteristic of MS, but instead showed an abnormality in the cerebellar folia. The CSF examination was consistent with an acute probable inflammatory cause and serology did not define an infectious cause. A cerebellar biopsy ruled out neoplastic and other causes. A follow-up brain MRI confirmed subsequent isolated cerebellar involvement with severe atrophy.

Case 47: An older gentleman with progressive gait ataxia and an abnormal brain MRI

A 69-year-old gentleman presented with a one- to one-and-half-year history of slowly progressive gait instability and personality changes. He started to

develop problems, suffering from falls which always occurred while he was doing something active, such as lifting heavy items or mowing the lawn. He said that he feels like he is going to fall and that he cannot catch himself. He reports no worsened problems when walking in the dark. He has had occasional anger outbursts, which his wife says was very unusual since he has always been very laid back. He had not displayed any dream enactment behavior or nocturnal stridor. One month of oral corticosteroid therapy did not produce any improvement in the symptoms.

On examination there was no significant orthostatic hypotension. He scored 33/38 on a Kokmen short test of mental status. His speech was dysarthric and of a mixed ataxic, spastic and hypophonic character. A motor exam was found to be normal, as were reflexes with bilateral flexor plantar responses. He had moderate vibratory loss in the distal bilateral lower extremities. He had mild bilateral appendicular ataxia with a wide-based ataxic gait.

A brain MRI showed symmetrical T2 signal abnormality involving the middle cerebellar peduncles bilaterally with mild atrophy of the midbrain, medulla and cerebellum (Figure 7.4). A CSF examination was normal. Serum testing for Lyme and paraneoplastic disorders was negative. Genetic testing for dominantly

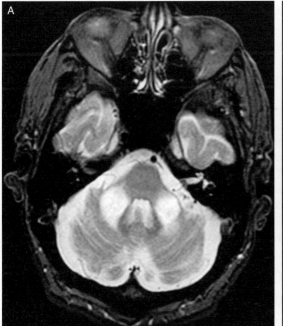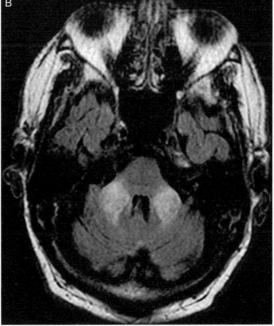

Figure 7.4 Axial T2 and FLAIR MRI brain demonstrates non-enhancing, symmetrical T2 signal abnormality involving the middle cerebellar peduncles bilaterally with mild atrophy of the midbrain, medulla and cerebellum.

inherited spinocerebellar ataxias was negative. Further testing showed an abnormality of the FMR-1 gene. An expanded CGG repeat of 88 was detected, indicating he is a carrier of Fragile X syndrome. Southern blot analysis suggested a normal methylation pattern. The finding of 88 CGG repeats and normal methylation pattern suggests the presence of a premutation within the Fragile X gene.

Three-step assessment

1 Classical clinical features of MS: progressive cerebellar ataxia with cognitive disorder.
2 Neurological examination: cerebellar ataxia, vibratory sense reduction
3 Investigations: MRI brain not consistent with MS; CSF not consistent with MS; genetic testing diagnostic of Fragile X associated tremor ataxia syndrome (FXTAS)

   Diagnosis: Fragile X associated tremor ataxia syndrome (FXTAS).

   Tip: Individuals with premutation within the Fragile X gene (a small expansion of the causative gene) were originally thought to be asymptomatic. FXTAS syndrome has more recently been described with hallmark symptoms and signs of late-onset ataxia, tremor, Parkinsonism and memory loss. Characteristic, but not pathognomic, MRI features include bilateral, symmetrical T2 signal abnormality in the middle cerebellar peduncles as demonstrated in this case, often with atrophy. There is no treatment for FXTAS other than symptomatic therapy.

Case 48: An older woman with progressive ataxia, urinary symptoms, an abnormal brain MRI and a family history of MS

A 64-year-old woman presented with a three-year history of progressive gait unsteadiness. She began to use a walker two years ago and one year ago she required a wheelchair for longer distances and currently could only take a few steps with bilateral assistance. She denied having memory loss and had no visual symptoms. She reported gradually worsening dysarthria and dysphagia to liquids and solids. She has urgency-related incontinence, double voiding and hesitancy without any bowel symptoms. She described feeling lightheaded when both sitting and standing. The patient's mother and a distant cousin have MS but there was no family history of cerebellar ataxia.

On neurological examination her mental status was found to be normal. Extraocular movements showed gaze-evoked nystagmus with a saccadic breakdown of pursuit eye movements. There was no palatal tremor (myoclonus). Motor power was normal, stretch reflexes were symmetrical and plantar responses were flexor bilaterally. She was essentially wheelchair bound with severe truncal and appendicular ataxia with appendicular dysmetria.

A brain MRI showed scattered non-specific foci of T2/FLAIR hyperintensity which was greater in the left basal ganglia region and white matter of both cerebral hemispheres without enhancement. Atrophic changes were seen of the cerebellum, pons and medulla which were out of proportion to normal-appearing cerebral hemispheres with a "hot cross bun" sign (Figure 7.5 A). Autonomic studies showed moderately severe adrenergic dysfunction, with cardiovagal and postganglionic sudomotor functions preserved, which were highly suggestive of a central autonomic disorder. A thermoregulatory sweat test showed anhidrosis of trunk and lower extremities consistent with central autonomic disorder such as multiple systems atrophy (Figure 7.5 B).

Three-step assessment

1 Classical clinical features of MS: progressive cerebellar ataxia
2 Neurological examination: severe cerebellar ataxia
3 Investigations: MRI brain not consistent with MS; autonomic studies and thermoregulatory sweat test consistent with multiple systems atrophy

   Diagnosis: Multiple systems atrophy cerebellar type (MSA-C).

   Tip: The important diagnostic clues here were the progressive and severe nature of the cerebellar ataxia and autonomic disorder. This was despite the lack of signs of corticospinal tract dysfunction (upper motor neuron weakness, extensor plantar responses). The MRI brain appearance with T2 changes not suggestive of MS and the brainstem atrophy with corresponding "hot-cross bun" sign are consistent with MSA-C. The significant findings on objective autonomic testing are consistent with MSA-C.

Case 49: A woman with a history of lymphoma and Sjögren syndrome with progressive ataxia

A 67-year-old woman presented with gait ataxia of uncertain etiology. The patient had a long history of

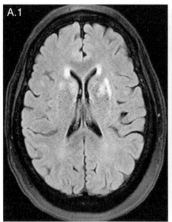
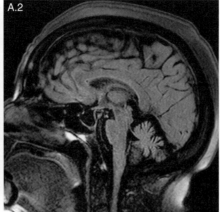
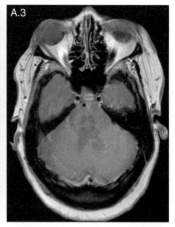

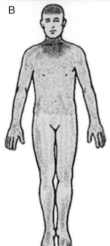

RESULTS

Oral temp before: **35.4** $^{\circ}$C after: **37.8** $^{\circ}$C

%anhid: **85.7**

Distribution: **MIXED**

IMPRESSION

There was patchy hypo/anhidrosis over most of the trunk and lower limbs. These findings can be seen in central autonomic disorders such as MSA.

Figure 7.5 A) 1, 2, 3 Axial T2 and FLAIR and Sagittal FLAIR MRI brain showing scattered, non-enhancing, non-specific foci of T2/FLAIR hyperintensity involving the left basal ganglia region more than the right, and white matter of both cerebral hemispheres. Atrophic changes of cerebellum, pons and medulla are out of proportion to normal-appearing cerebral hemispheres and demonstrate the "hot-cross bun" sign. B) Thermoregulatory sweat test shows anhidrosis of trunk and lower extremities consistent with central autonomic disorder such as multiple systems atrophy.

recurrent and treatment-resistant MALT lymphoma, as well as a history of Sjögren syndrome requiring immunosuppressive treatment with rituximab. She reported gait ataxia and incoordination and dysarthria worsening over the last few months. She would stumble to the right more than the left and required a walking stick but continued to fall. She had no mental status changes, weakness, dysphagia, pain or sensory loss.

Her mental status and visual fields were normal. Her extraocular movements revealed saccadic pursuit extraocular movements with impaired suppression of the vestibulo-ocular reflex. There was no palatal myoclonus. She had significant cerebellar-type dysarthria. Her motor exam was normal and plantar responses were flexor. She had action tremor that was greater on her right side, with incoordination of the lower

extremities also greater on the right than left and marked gait ataxia.

A brain MRI showed areas of abnormal T2 signal within the middle cerebellar peduncles with significant cerebellar atrophy and gadolinium enhancement in the cerebellar folia and the cerebellar vermis (Figure 7.6). A CSF examination showed a normal white blood cell count, protein and glucose with four unique oligoclonal bands and was negative for malignancy. A CSF JC virus PCR was positive.

Three-step analysis

1 Classical clinical features of MS: progressive cerebellar ataxia
2 Neurological examination: consistent with cerebellar disease

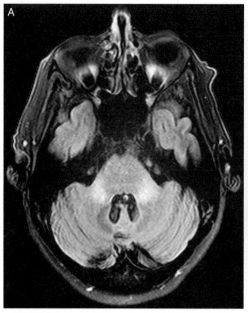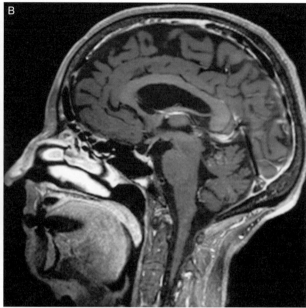

Figure 7.6 Sagittal T1 with a gadolinium MRI head shows cerebellar atrophy, with gadolinium enhancement in the folia of the anterior-superior cerebellar vermis. Increased T2 signal was also observed in the same distribution (not shown).

3 Investigations: MRI brain not consistent with MS; CSF JC virus PCR positive

Diagnosis: Progressive multifocal leukoencephalopathy (PML) infection of the cerebellar granule cell layer.

Tip: PML may in rare cases affect the cerebellar granule cells and cause a severe cerebellar impairment rather than typical multifocal cerebral white matter disease. Although there are no known cures for PML, the patient initiated treatment for a JC virus infection with cytosine arabinoside.

Further reading

Agnihotri SP, Dang X, Carter JL, et al. JCV GCN in a natalizumab-treated MS patient is associated with mutations of the VP1 capsid gene. *Neurology* 2014;**83**: 727–32.

Dang L, Dang X, Koralnik IJ, Todd PK. JC polyomavirus granule cell neuronopathy in a patient treated with rituximab. *JAMA Neurol* 2014;**71**:487–9.

Dang X, Vidal JE, Oliveira AC, et al. JC virus granule cell neuronopathy is associated with VP1 C terminus mutants. *J Gen Virol* 2012;**93**:175–83.

Deguchi K, Ikeda K, Kume K, et al. Significance of the hot-cross bun sign on T2*-weighted MRI for the diagnosis of multiple system atrophy. *J Neurol* 2015.

Di Donato I, Banchi S, Federico A, Dotti MT. Adult-onset genetic leukoencephalopathies.

Focus on the more recently defined forms. *Curr Mol Med* 2014.

Dirven CM, Mooij JJ, Molenaar WM. Cerebellar pilocytic astrocytoma: a treatment protocol based upon analysis of 73 cases and a review of the literature. *Childs Nerv Syst* 1997;**13**:17–23.

Filley CM, Brown MS, Onderko K, et al. White matter disease and cognitive impairment in FMR1 premutation carriers. *Neurology* 2015.

Hagerman PJ, Hagerman RJ. Fragile X-associated tremor/ataxia syndrome. *Ann N Y Acad Sci* 2015;**1338**:58–70.

Lin DJ, Hermann KL, Schmahmann JD. Multiple system atrophy of the cerebellar type: clinical state of the art. *Mov Disord* 2014;**29**:294–304.

Mascalchi M, Vella A. Magnetic resonance and nuclear medicine imaging in ataxias. *Handb Clin Neurol* 2012;**103**:85–110.

Pruitt AA. Infections of the cerebellum. *Neurol Clin* 2014;**32**:1117–31.

Sasaki T, Saito R, Kumabe T, et al. Transformation of adult cerebellar pilocytic astrocytoma to glioblastoma. *Brain Tumor pathol* 2014;**31**:108–12.

Wade A, Hayhurst C, Amato-Watkins A, Lammie A, Leach P. Cerebellar pilocytic astrocytoma in adults: a management paradigm for a rare tumour. *Acta Neurochir (Wien)* 2013;**155**:1431–5.

Ye JM, Ye MJ, Kranz S, Lo P. A 10 year retrospective study of surgical outcomes of adult intracranial pilocytic astrocytoma. *J Clin Neurosci* 2014;**21**:2160–4.

Challenges in diagnosing demyelinating brainstem disease

The brainstem is a relatively small area of the CNS that contains critical, phylogenetically old structures. Symptoms of brainstem dysfunction indicate impairment of the connections with the cerebellum (ataxia) as well as impairment of the cranial nerve connections (e.g. diplopia, facial sensory loss and vertigo). Signs of brainstem dysfunction, including internuclear ophthalmoplegia, nystagmus, quadriparesis, coma, locked-in syndrome and gait and limb ataxia, may be paramount in evaluating MS. Mimickers of MS may herald similar features of brainstem dysfunction and need to be assessed prior to diagnosing MS.

Case 50: A woman with diplopia and transient right arm incoordination

A 38-year-old woman presented having gone through a one- to one-and-half-week episode of painless binocular diplopia. After that, she had a sudden onset of dysarthria and right upper and lower extremity incoordination. That symptom lasted only ten minutes before resolving itself and it was not repetitive. She was initially evaluated for a possible stroke. She had not had other clinical attacks of multiple sclerosis or neurological impairment before. The patient's maternal second cousin has multiple sclerosis.

On neurological examination, her mental status was found to be normal. Extraocular movements were intact with no internuclear ophthalmoplegia or nystagmus. Her speech was clear and a motor exam was normal throughout. Her reflexes were intact and plantar responses were flexor bilaterally. Her gait and coordination were also intact.

A brain MRI showed multiple areas of abnormal T2 signal with a large enhancing lesion in the midbrain consistent with MS (Figure 8.1). A cervical spine MRI showed a couple of lesions consistent with MS. A thoracic spine MRI was not performed. A CSF showed elevated oligoclonal bands and IgG index.

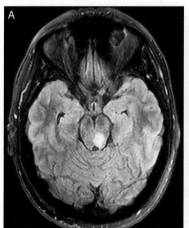 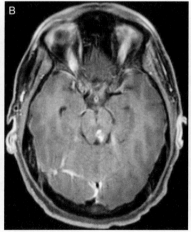 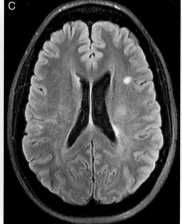

Figure 8.1 Axial FLAIR and T1 with gadolinium MRI brain shows abnormal signal within the left tegmentum of the pons with patchy peripheral enhancement without mass effect, with scattered T2 hyperintensity in the periventricular deep white matter of both hemispheres consistent with multiple sclerosis with active brainstem demyelination.

Three-step assessment

1 Classical clinical features of MS: painless binocular diplopia, asymmetrical limb incoordination
2 Neurological examination: normal
3 Investigations: MRI brain consistent with MS; MRI cervical spinal cord MRI consistent with MS; CSF consistent with MS

Diagnosis: Relapsing remitting multiple sclerosis.

Tip: Occasionally symptoms of demyelination may have a sudden onset and brief duration, thereby mimicking a cerebrovascular cause. Evaluations in this patient revealed additional evidence of demyelination in the brain and cervical spinal cord as well as CSF abnormalities consistent with MS.

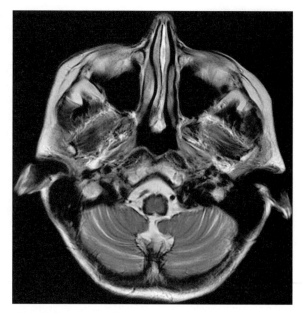

Figure 8.2 Axial FLAIR MRI brain shows T2 hypointensity surrounding an atrophic brainstem and into cerebellar folia consistent with superficial siderosis.

Case 51: Progressive gait impairment in a woman on chronic anticoagulation therapy

A 64-year-old woman presented with progressive numbness, weakness and gait ataxia over the prior two and half years. She recalled initially developing numbness in the left foot which progressed up the left lower extremity and then involved the right lower extremity. She had no cognitive impairment or hearing loss. She started to use a cane and then a walker, but despite that continued to experience falls.

On neurological examination, her visual fields and extraocular movements were normal. She had moderate quadriparesis in the upper and lower extremities. Her reflexes were intact in the upper extremities and markedly reduced in the lower extremities with bilateral extensor plantar responses. There was severe, multiple modality sensory loss in the lower extremities. She had also severe gait impairment and needed bilateral assistance to stand.

Brain, cervical and thoracic spine MRIs showed no evidence of MS but did show hemosiderin deposit throughout (Figure 8.2). A CSF examination showed a white cell count of 40 with 712 red blood cells and marked xanthochromia. CSF protein was elevated at 83 mg/dL, while her oligoclonal bands, IgG index NMO-IgG and paraneoplastic autoantibody screen were all normal. Serological testing for NMO-IgG antibodies, ferritin, and angiotensin converting enzyme (ACE) were all normal.

Three-step assessment

1 Classical clinical features of MS: progressive myelopathy with gait ataxia
2 Neurological examination: consistent with myelopathy
3 Investigations: brain, spinal cord MRI negative for MS but consistent with other neurological disease – superficial siderosis; CSF consistent with superficial siderosis

Diagnosis: Superficial siderosis.

Tip: A typical clinical presentation of superficial siderosis is an older patient with risk factors for bleeding. A typical presentation would be hearing loss, dementia and significant ataxia. It is important to look for siderosis to rule out changes of primary progressive multiple sclerosis as a cause for significant progressive gait impairment.

Case 52: A young man with personality change, ataxia and progressive brain white matter changes

A 20-year-old gentleman presented with significant personality change and ataxia over a number of years. He was the product of a normal pregnancy and

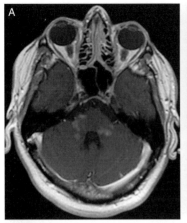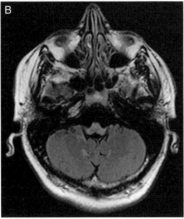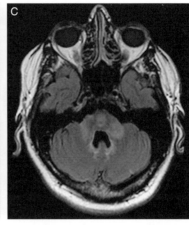

Figure 8.3 Axial FLAIR and T1 with gadolinium MRI brain shows confluent areas of abnormal T2 hyperintensity involving the central pons, middle cerebellar peduncles, dentate nuclei and medulla with associated patchy enhancement, particularly of the cerebellar peduncle and medullary lesions with marked medullary atrophy.

delivery and met his early developmental milestones as expected. By fourth grade he was declining academically, and by sixth grade he had incoordination and imbalance. In his teenage years he had impaired judgment and problems with impulse control, resulting in his being fired from his job for socially inappropriate behavior. He developed dysphagia and hypernasal speech and became progressively less intelligible. A paternal uncle had multiple sclerosis and his maternal great-grandfather had amyotrophic lateral sclerosis (ALS).

On neurological examination, he was short in stature with a head circumference of 58.0 cm (normal adult head circumference is 55.9 cm with a standard deviation of 1.85 cm). He scored 31 out of 38 on a short test of mental status. He had horizontal gaze-evoked nystagmus with evidence of palatal myoclonus (palatal tremor). His motor power was normal as was his sensation, but his tandem walking was ataxic.

A brain MRI showed multiple areas of abnormal T2 signal in the white matter diffusely and confluent with a frontal predominance (not shown). Importantly, there was significant atrophy of the medulla and pons with signal abnormality (Figure 8.3). There was persistent gadolinium enhancement involving the cerebellar peduncle on the right side. Genetic testing confirmed evidence of a mutation in the glial fibrillary acidic protein (GFAP) gene, confirming Alexander disease.

Three-step assessment

1 Classical clinical features of MS: progressive cognitive and brainstem dysfunction

2 Neurological examination: ataxia and cognitive impairment with palatal myoclonus (palatal tremor), macrocephaly

3 Investigations: brain, spinal cord MRI negative for MS; consistent with other neurological disease – genetic testing confirmed mutation in the glial fibrillary acidic protein (GFAP) diagnostic of Alexander disease

Diagnosis: Alexander disease.

Tip: The key diagnostic points in this case are of a frontal predominant white matter disease with severe medullary atrophy and enhancement. The evidence of palatal myoclonus on examination, as well as the ataxia, is consistent with Alexander disease. Some patients presenting in adulthood may not have macrocephaly. The GFAP mutation analysis is diagnostic, as it was in this case.

Case 53: A young man with rapidly progressive impairment and brainstem hemorrhage

A 20-year-old man, who was otherwise well and with no prior medical illnesses, presented with acute onset of lower extremity paresthesias, painless binocular diplopia, gait ataxia, left facial weakness and dysarthria. He had no prodromal constitutional symptoms and no fever, headache, ill contacts, or recent travel. His symptoms rapidly worsened over days; he suffered from progressive respiratory compromise and required mechanical ventilation.

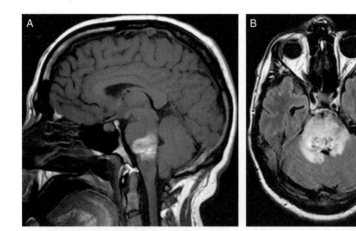
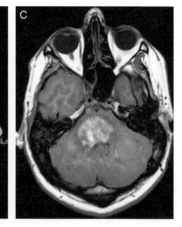

Figure 8.4 Sagittal T1 without gadolinium, Axial FLAIR and T1 with gadolinium MRI brain shows extensive area of increased T1 and decreased T2 signal consistent with subacute hemorrhage, increased T2 signal with an irregular ring of enhancement, with mass effect in the pons, and extension of signal abnormality into the middle cerebellar peduncles.

On neurological examination he was intubated and sedated with quadriparesis and an essentially "locked-in" state.

He was treated with corticosteroids, plasma exchange and intravenous cyclophosphamide but did not respond and died soon after.

Serial brain MRIs showed a progressively enlarging area of abnormal T2 signal within the brainstem with gadolinium enhancement. Progressive expansion of the lesion and ring enhancement was then associated with subtle subacute hemorrhage. A subsequent brain MRI demonstrated severe necrosis with gross hemorrhage (Figure 8.4). Cervical and thoracic spine MRIs were both normal as was a brain MR angiography. A CSF examination showed 25 white blood cells (51 percent monocytes, 41 percent lymphocytes). Protein was elevated at 70 mg/dL. His IgG index was elevated to 1.64, but there were no unique CSF oligoclonal bands. Tests for infectious agents, including listeria, fungal, bacterial, microbacterial cultures, herpes simplex virus, varicella zoster virus, cytomegalovirus, Epstein-Barr virus, human herpesvirus 6 and Whipple's agent polymerase chain reaction (PCR), were all negative. The autopsy confirmed evidence of a hemorrhagic necrotizing inflammatory process consistent with acute hemorrhagic leukoencephalitis (Hurst) disease.

Three-step assessment

1   Classical clinical features of MS: acute progressive brainstem dysfunction; severe, treatment resistant

2   Neurological examination: progressive findings of severe brainstem dysfunction with respiratory compromise

3   Investigations: brain MRI: severe demyelinating disease with hemorrhage; spinal cord MRI: negative for MS; CSF consistent with CNS demyelinating cause; autopsy confirmed acute hemorrhagic leukoencephalitis (Hurst) disease

Diagnosis: Acute hemorrhagic leukoencephalitis (Hurst) disease

Tip: Hurst disease is regarded as a severe form of acute disseminated encephalomyelitis. Treatment is with corticosteroids and plasma exchange. However, some cases are so severe they do not respond to this therapy. Hemorrhage is often petechial and disseminated but may be gross and focal, as demonstrated in this case.

Case 54:   A man with facial tingling, ataxia and brainstem predominant perivascular enhancement on brain MRI

A 37-year-old gentleman presented with a two-year history of intermittent facial tingling. He then developed painless horizontal binocular diplopia with gait ataxia worsening over a number of months. An MRI showed evidence of subtle T2 signal abnormality but enhanced T1 imaging showed a more prominent, unusual, pepper-like gadolinium enhancement in the brainstem, particularly prominent in the pons.

He was treated with five days of intravenous methyl-prednisolone with marked improvement and had resolution of his symptoms for one year and prompt, but incomplete, improvement in the MRI findings; however, these symptoms recurred along with worsened gait ataxia, dysarthria and diplopia. He reinitiated corticosteroids but on tapering oral prednisone therapy, he reliably worsened clinically with a recurrence of the abnormal MRI findings. He was then treated chronically with corticosteroids and methotrexate. After many years, he became stable clinically and radiologically on immunosuppressive monotherapy with methotrexate.

On neurological examination his mental status was found to be normal but he had some pseudobulbar affect heralded by uncontrollable laughter. Extraocular movements showed gaze evoked nystagmus and he had a cerebellar dysarthria. He had no motor weakness and his reflexes were intact, with bilateral extensor plantar responses. He had incoordination of both upper and lower extremities and his gait was ataxic.

A brain MRI showed areas of abnormal T2 signal with perivascular gadolinium enhancement in the pons (Figure 8.5). Enlarging areas of gadolinium enhancement of the brainstem and cerebellum as well as similar perivascular lesions on MRI of the cervical and thoracic spinal cord were found. A CSF examination revealed elevated oligoclonal bands. A pontine brain biopsy was performed, which showed a chronic inflammatory disease without findings of infection, neoplasm, multiple sclerosis, sarcoidosis, lymphomatoid granulomatosis or histiocytosis.

Three-step assessment

1 Classical clinical features of MS: chronic, relapsing brainstem symptoms, responsive to corticosteroids and immunosuppressive medications

2 Neurological examination: findings of brainstem, cerebellar and spinal cord dysfunction

3 Investigations: brain MRI – T2 abnormalities predominantly in the pons with perivascular gadolinium enhancement; spinal cord MRI – similar perivascular gadolinium enhancement; CSF consistent with CNS autoimmune disease; biopsy showed chronic inflammation without demyelination, infection or granulomatous disease consistent with chronic lymphocytic inflammation with pontine perivascular enhancement responsive to steroids (CLIPPERS).

Diagnosis: Chronic lymphocytic inflammation with pontine perivascular enhancement responsive to steroids (CLIPPERS).

Tip: This patient has features of a recently described syndrome termed "chronic lymphocytic inflammation with pontine perivascular enhancement responsive to steroids" (CLIPPERS). This is an inflammatory, possibly immune-mediated process with predominance in the brainstem. Numerous other patients have now been diagnosed with this condition since the initial paper describing this syndrome. Rare patients have been reported to develop malignancies, such as lymphoma, but the vast majority of patients remain having an inflammatory process that is often responsive to corticosteroids or other immunosuppressive treatments.

Case 55: A young woman with intractable vomiting

An 18-year-old woman was initially evaluated for intractable vomiting by a gastroenterologist. She required hospitalization for dehydration due to intractable vomiting for 10 to 15 days. An endoscopy was performed which revealed gastritis. The nausea

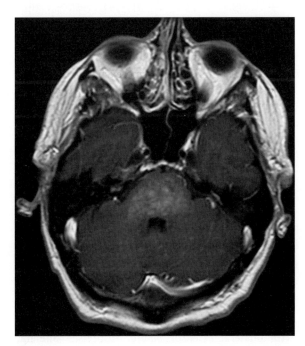

Figure 8.5 Axial FLAIR and T1 with gadolinium MRI brain shows T2 signal abnormality in the brain stem, with more marked perivascular enhancement within the mid pons extending into the middle cerebellar peduncles.

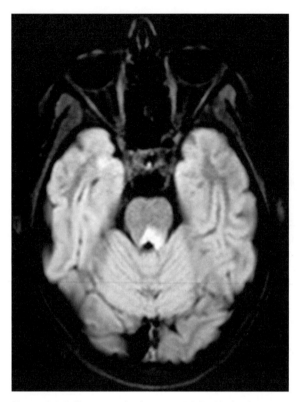

Figure 8.6 Diffusion weighted imaging MRI brain scan shows restricted diffusion around the pontine tegmentum and periaqueductal grey area due to neuromyelitis spectrum disorder.

improved but she continued to vomit once per week. She had a history of joint pain involving the knees, ankles, wrists and fingers. A serum antinuclear antibody (ANA) was strongly positive. An initial brain MRI was felt to be normal. Three months later she developed binocular painless diplopia and a repeat MRI showed more definite lesions in the brainstem and high cervical spinal cord. The patient's neurological examination was entirely normal. A brain MRI showed a number of T2 lesions in the periependymal regions of the brainstem and the floor of the fourth ventricle extending from the midbrain into the medulla (Figure 8.6). In addition, there was a ventral medullary lesion and a lesion on the left side of the cervical cord at C1. The supratentorial white matter was normal. NMO-IgG serology aquaporin-4 test was positive.

Three-step assessment

1 Classical clinical features of MS: none typical
2 Neurological examination: normal
3 Investigations: brain MRI: negative for MS; area postrema lesion consistent with other neurological

disease – neuromyelitis optica spectrum disease; CSF normal; Serology NMO-IgG antibodies consistent with neuromyelitis optica spectrum disease

Diagnosis: Neuromyelitis optica spectrum disorder causing intractable vomiting.

Tip: Intractable vomiting may be a presenting episode of NMO spectrum disorders. Inflammatory changes are described in the area postrema and the medullary floor of the fourth ventricle areas enriched with aquaporin 4 water channels and without an intact blood brain barrier. Presentation to gastroenterologists is common and the vomiting is often severe and protracted.

Case 56: A woman of Ashkenazi Jewish heritage with a progressive gait disorder and abnormal brain and spine MRI

This 63-year-old woman had suffered from fatigue and gait imbalance for "most of her life," and had always walked slowly and had difficulty ice skating. Her gait impairment was noticed by her family members about 15 years prior to presentation and had been an insidious, slowly progressive gait disorder since then. She required a cane four years prior to presentation, then a walker two years prior, and then a scooter one year ago. She had symptoms of neurogenic bladder dysfunction with bladder frequency and urge-related incontinence over the prior 15 years which had also slowly worsened.

She reported never having any attack-like worsening such as optic neuritis or acute brainstem problems. She had no constitutional or systemic symptoms apart from dry mouth, which was attributed to medications. She had no history of tobacco, alcohol, or illicit drug use. Her background was Ashkenazi Jewish, with no known family history of neurological disease.

On neurological examination, her mental status was normal, as were her cranial nerves and motor examination in the face and upper extremities. She had severe symmetrical weakness in the lower extremities bilaterally in an upper motor neuron pyramidal distribution. Her reflexes were symmetrically brisk with bilateral extensor plantar responses. She had sensory deficit to pinpricks and temperature bilaterally up to her knees. Her gait was severely spastic and ataxic, requiring a walker.

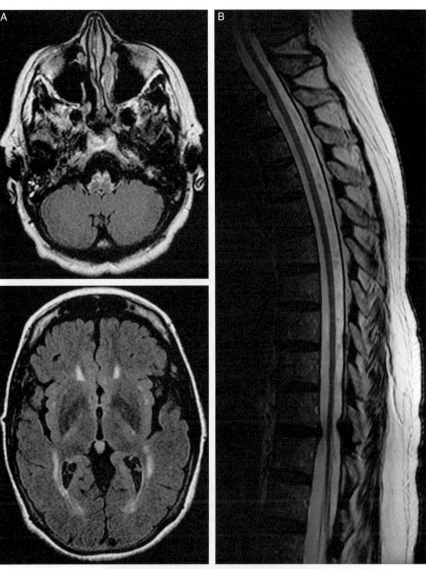

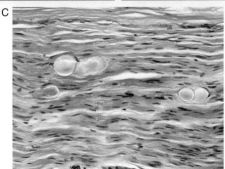

Figure 8.7 A) Axial FLAIR MRI brain scan shows bilaterally symmetric, non-enhancing T2 signal abnormality involving the periphery of the cervicomedullary junction extending superiorly into the medulla. At the midbrain level, there was signal abnormality laterally with contiguous signal abnormality extending into the cerebral peduncles (not shown). Scattered non-specific foci of T2 signal hyperintensity are seen in the hemispheric white matter bilaterally. B) Sagittal T2 MRI thoracic spinal cord demonstrates symmetrical atrophy throughout that was also seen in the cervical spinal cord (not shown). C) Sural nerve biopsy showed multiple round PAS positive intraneural figures are present consistent with polyglucosan bodies.

A brain MRI scan showed T2 signal abnormality involving the brainstem, superior cerebellar peduncles and periventricular region without gadolinium enhancement or restricted diffusion (Figure 8.7 A). Cervical and thoracic spinal cord MRIs showed atrophy with cord signal abnormality centrally and at the dorsal cord throughout the cervical region (Figure 8.7 B). A CSF examination showed 10 white blood cells, protein 47, with no elevations in oligoclonal bands or IgG index. Nerve conduction studies showed low amplitude motor responses and a low amplitude sural sensory response, without temporal dispersion or conduction block. An electromyography showed fibrillation potentials and very poor activation, with long duration and high amplitude potentials consistent with an axonal polyneuropathy with a superimposed central nervous system process accounting for the poor activation. A sural nerve biopsy showed multiple polyglucosan bodies (Figure 8.7 C). Skin fibroblasts showed reduced branching enzyme activity suggestive of glycogen storage disease type IV, which is consistent with Adult Onset Polyglucosan Body Disease.

Three-step assessment

1 Classical clinical features of MS: progressive gait ataxia and upper motor neuron weakness with neurogenic bladder dysfunction

2 Neurological examination: consistent with myelopathy

3 Investigations: brain MRI inconsistent with MS; spinal cord MRI inconsistent with MS but consistent with other neurological disease; CSF normal; EMG consistent with axonal peripheral neuropathy sural nerve biopsy and skin fibroblast branching enzyme deficiency diagnostic of polyglucosan body disease

Diagnosis: Adult onset polyglucosan body disease.

Tip: Adult onset polyglucosan body disease typically presents in the fifth or sixth decade and is more common among the Ashkenazi Jewish population. It is slowly progressive, an autosomal recessive disorder allelic to type IV glycogen storage disease with glycogen branching enzyme mutations. Early neurogenic bladder involvement, occasionally with cognitive impairment, is common with electrophysiological evidence of axonal polyneuropathy.

Brain MRIs, as in this case, show symmetrical white matter abnormalities with brainstem abnormalities, and spinal MRIs show diffuse cord atrophy. A CSF examination should not show markers of autoimmune disease such as elevated oligoclonal bands or IgG index, as was the case here.

Further reading

Abou Zeid NE, Burns JD, Wijdicks EF, Giannini C, Keegan BM. Atypical acute hemorrhagic leukoencephalitis (Hurst's disease) presenting with focal hemorrhagic brainstem lesion. *Neurocritical care* 2010;**12**:95–7.

Pittock SJ, Debruyne J, Krecke KN, et al. Chronic lymphocytic inflammation with pontine perivascular enhancement responsive to steroids (CLIPPERS). *Brain* 2010;**133**:2626–34.

Lossos A, Klein CJ, McEvoy KM, Keegan BM. A 63-year-old woman with urinary incontinence and progressive gait disorder. *Neurology* 2009;**72**:1607–13.

Mochel F, Schiffmann R, Steenweg ME, et al. Adult polyglucosan body disease: Natural History and Key Magnetic Resonance Imaging Findings. *Ann Neurol* 2012;**72**:433–41.

Paradas C, Akman HO, Ionete C, et al. Branching enzyme deficiency: expanding the clinical spectrum. *JAMA Neurol* 2014;**71**:41–7.

Limousin N, Praline J, Motica O, et al. Brain biopsy is required in steroid-resistant patients with chronic lymphocytic inflammation with pontine perivascular enhancement responsive to steroids (CLIPPERS). *J Neurooncol* 2012;**107**:223–4.

Simon NG, Parratt JD, Barnett MH, et al. Expanding the clinical, radiological and neuropathological phenotype of chronic lymphocytic inflammation with pontine perivascular enhancement responsive to steroids (CLIPPERS). *J Neurol Neurosurg Psychiatry* 2012;**83**:15–22.

Lekgabe E, Kavar B. Progression and management of superficial siderosis. *J Clin Neurosci* 2012;**19**:906–8.

Vale TC, Gomez RS, Teixeira AL. Idiopathic superficial siderosis. *Arch Neurol* 2011;**68**:1334–5.

Kumar N. Neuroimaging in superficial siderosis: an in-depth look. *AJNR Am J Neuroradiol* 2010;**31**:5–14.

Kumar N, Cohen-Gadol AA, Wright RA, Miller GM, Piepgras DG, Ahlskog JE. Superficial siderosis. *Neurology* 2006;**66**:1144–52.

Apiwattanakul M, Popescu BF, Matiello M, et al. Intractable vomiting as the initial presentation of neuromyelitis optica. *Ann Neurol* 2010;**68**:757–61.

Popescu BF, Lennon VA, Parisi JE, et al. Neuromyelitis optica unique area postrema lesions: nausea, vomiting, and pathogenic implications. *Neurology* 2011;**76**:1229–37.

Challenges in diagnosing spinal cord disease

MS patients frequently present with symptoms of an inflammatory spinal cord sensory-level, upper motor neuron paraparesis or quadriparesis, as well as bowel and bladder dysfunction. Importantly, the most common presentation of primary and secondary progressive forms of MS is of insidiously progressive gait disorder due to progressive myelopathy. This progressive impairment is usually identified on clinical history with functional ambulatory impairment occurring earlier and earlier, with the patient able to exert themselves less and less over months to years. An individual may report walking for many miles a few years ago, and over time come to have worsening, often asymmetrical leg weakness so that impairment arises over one mile, then after half a mile, and then even shorter distances over time. Inherited, nutritional, vascular, compressive, infectious and other inflammatory etiologies may affect the spinal cord to mimic both acute MS attacks as well as progressive MS–related myelopathy.

Case 57: A patient with an abnormal brain MRI scan and cervical spine lesion. Is it MS?

A woman fell 15 years prior to presentation, suffering bruises. Ten years prior to presentation, she developed numbness in the right fourth and fifth digits with tingling paresthesias and weakness in her right lower extremity. A cervical spine MRI showed cervical spondylosis with an area of intramedullary abnormal T2 signal at the area of compression. She underwent a cervical spine laminectomy which led to improvement in the hand's paresthesias, but she remained with right-sided leg weakness.

She was referred for the possibility of secondary progressive multiple sclerosis given abnormalities found on brain and spinal cord MRIs. Her clinical history was clear, however, that she had experienced no progressive weakness, numbness or gait

impairment involving the right lower extremity or elsewhere over the intervening seven years, and this was confirmed by her husband. Correspondingly, she used no gait aids and only rarely fell.

She had no prior classical clinical features of attacks of multiple sclerosis including optic neuritis, diplopia, dysarthria, dysphagia, hemiparesis, hemisensory deficit or symptoms of a resolving sensory myelopathy. There was no family history of multiple sclerosis, and she had hypertension and a 30-pack-per-year history of cigarette smoking. A neurological examination was consistent only with signs of an asymmetrical cervical myelopathy with impairment on the right side.

A brain MRI showed multiple, non-specific areas of non-enhancing abnormal T2 signal randomly throughout the cerebral white matter. A cervical spine MRI scan showed a subtle area of non-enhancing increased T2 signal as well as postoperative changes from the decompressive surgery (Figure 9.1). A preoperative cervical spinal MRI showed a compressive lesion around the area of abnormal signal. A thoracic spine MRI was normal. A CSF showed no elevations in IgG index or oligoclonal bands. Visual evoked potentials and somatosensory evoked potentials were normal.

Three-step assessment

1 Classical clinical features of MS: none, static non-progressive myelopathy associated with prior compressive trauma
2 Neurological examination: consistent with myelopathy
3 Investigations: brain MRI – non-specific; spinal cord MRI – myelomalacia from old trauma; CSF normal; evoked potentials normal

Diagnosis: Static cervical myelopathy due to old compression but no evidence of progressive multiple sclerosis.

Tip: The only way to identify progressive forms of multiple sclerosis is on history and on examination.

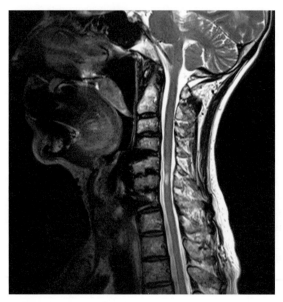

Figure 9.1 Sagittal T2 MRI cervical spine shows a solitary area of increased T2 signal at the prior level of compression, now relieved by spinal decompressive surgery.

On neurological examination, her mental status, cranial nerve and motor examination in the face and upper extremities were normal. She had severe weakness in a pyramidal distribution on the right lower extremity only. Plantar responses were extensor on the right and equivocal on the left. She walked with a right-sided circumductive upper motor neuron weakness gait. Vibratory sense was minimally reduced in the toes.

A brain MRI showed lesions highly suggestive of MS. Upon reviewing the outside cervical spinal MRI, the initial cervical spondylotic changes did not show an area of abnormal signal at the level of most severe compression (Figure 9.2). There was, however, an area of abnormal T2 signal in the high cervical cord that was clearly separate from the area of spinal cord compression. Additionally, a thoracic spine MRI showed areas of abnormal T2 signal consistent with MS. A CSF examination was undertaken and was found to be normal. She had never had visual evoked potentials.

This patient had no clear clinical history of progressive myelopathic symptoms over a number of years. She had a static myelopathy entirely related to an old compressive lesion. The areas of abnormal signal on the MRI scan were non-specific and not characteristic of MS. Importantly, other tests looking for evidence of multiple sclerosis were normal, including an MRI scan of the thoracic spine, a CSF examination and evoked potentials.

Case 58: A woman with continued progressive gait impairment after successful cervical fusion surgery

A 52-year-old woman presented with a four-year history of progressive walking impairment. She had become limited to walking only a few blocks. A cervical spine MRI scan showed spondylotic changes. There was no significant pain, but local providers recommended spinal surgery and a cervical spinal fusion was performed two years prior to presentation. Despite the surgery, she continued to have worsened gait impairment over time. She had impaired bladder emptying on ultrasound evaluation. She had a history of type 2 diabetes mellitus, hyperlipidemia and hypertension. There was no family history of multiple sclerosis.

Three-step assessment

1 Classical clinical features of MS: progressive myelopathy
2 Neurological examination: consistent with myelopathy
3 Investigations: brain MRI consistent with MS; cervical spinal cord MRI – spondylotic changes but abnormal intramedullary cord lesion separate from compressive area consistent with MS; MRI thoracic spine consistent with MS; CSF normal

Diagnosis: Primary progressive multiple sclerosis.

Tip: Multiple sclerosis MRI spinal cord lesions may be subtle. If there are areas of stenosis due to cervical spondylosis, it should be assured that the most prominent area of intramedullary abnormal T2 signal related to the stenosis should be directly adjacent or immediately rostral to the stenosis. The later MRI scan of the brain showed areas of abnormal signal that were highly suggestive of multiple sclerosis, as did the MRI thoracic spine, which was a compelling finding in the absence of CSF abnormalities of significance such as elevated IgG index or oligoclonal bands in this patient.

The progressive worsening after successful fusion surgery suggested that that was not the original cause for the progressive myelopathy.

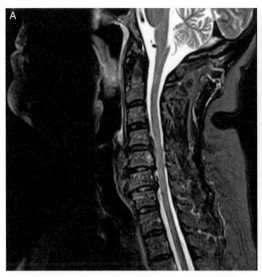
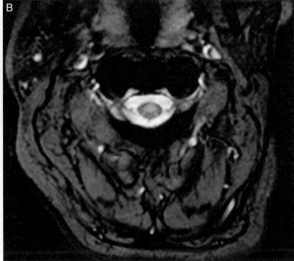

Figure 9.2 Sagittal and axial T2 MRI cervical spine shows demyelinating lesions within the cord parenchyma at C2 anteriorly, between C5 and C6 laterally and scattered throughout the thoracic cord (not shown) including a lesion within the conus. Postoperative changes of instrumented anterior interbody fusion with plate and screw fixation from the C4-C7 is demonstrated.

Case 59: Progressive hemiparesis in a man with a single cervical spinal cord lesion. Could this be MS?

A 58-year-old gentleman presented with progressive hemiparesis. He had noticed worsening left-sided weakness over the prior three years. He underwent lumbar spinal surgery for possible lumbar stenosis but he had no improvement. He had occasional paresthesias of the left hand and foot but did not have bowel or bladder impairment. When he lay supine he would get extensor spasms of the left lower extremity. He had no prominent fatigue but he required a cane to ambulate.

On examination, his mental status was found to be normal. His cranial nerves were also normal. He had moderate weakness in the left upper and lower extremities in a pyramidal distribution, with the right side being entirely normal. Reflexes were brisker on the left than on the right, and the plantar response was extensor on the left and equivocal on the right. He walked with a left-sided hemiparetic gait. His vibratory sense was impaired at the toes bilaterally.

A brain MRI showed a few areas of abnormal signal that were not highly suggestive of multiple sclerosis. A cervical spine MRI showed evidence of a single area of abnormal signal in the left lateral cord

at the C3-C4 level (Figure 9.3). A thoracic spine MRI was normal. A CSF examination showed the protein minimally elevated at 55 mg/dL and with nine unique oligoclonal bands. Serological evaluations were negative including vitamin B12, copper, ceruloplasmin, ANA, paraneoplastic autoantibody screen, HIV, Lyme screen, syphilis screen and very long-chain fatty acids. NMO-IgG antibodies were negative.

Three-step assessment

1 Classical clinical features of MS: progressive myelopathy
2 Neurological examination: consistent with myelopathy
3 Investigations: brain MRI not consistent with MS; cervical spinal cord MRI – single intramedullary cord lesion suggestive of MS; thoracic spinal cord MRI normal; CSF consistent with MS

Diagnosis: Solitary sclerosis presentation of primary progressive multiple sclerosis.

Tip: Patients may have a progressive myelopathy with only a single MRI lesion associated with the characteristic features of demyelination of multiple sclerosis. Progressive impairment may occur bilaterally if the single MRI lesion is large and it may cause quadriparesis when it is located in the cervicomedullary junction.

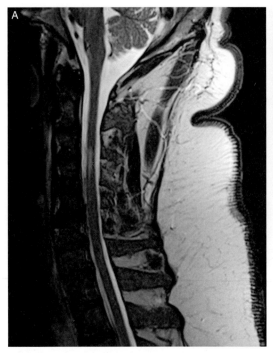
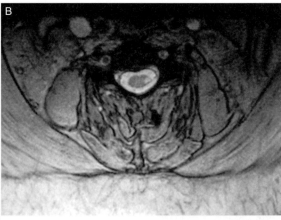

Figure 9.3 Sagittal and axial T2 MRI cervical spine showed abnormal T2 hyperintensity involving a left lateral aspect of cord at C3–4 level without associated cord expansion. Considerations include focus of demyelination such as related to MS.

Case 60: A man with gait impairment after bronchitis. Is it transverse myelitis?

A 76-year-old gentleman was well until four months prior to presentation. He had recovered from a viral upper respiratory tract infection on a trip to Alaska. He noticed, while riding his bike, that whenever he would hit a bump he would get a tingling sensation radiating down both upper extremities. He then developed a walking impairment with significant gait imbalance. The next month, while cutting down trees, he noticed a weakness in the upper extremities proximally and muscle stiffness. He was felt to have rotator cuff tendon disease, and underwent injections and physical therapy. Subsequently he developed tingling sensation of all fingers of both hands with numbness of the left greater than right foot. While he was previously active in the health club, he now could not lift the same amount of weights and he had difficulty even with activities such as tying his shoes, buttoning shirts and opening jars. He had no bowel or bladder incontinence. He noticed an aching sensation and a "tired" sensation in his neck.

He had no prior symptoms of clinical attacks of multiple sclerosis such as optic neuritis, diplopia, hemiparesis or hemisensory deficit in the past. He also had no history of symptoms of inflammatory myelopathy.

On neurological examination it was found that facial and proximal upper extremities power was normal. Weakness was found to be greater in the left than right wrist extensors, finger extensors and all intrinsic hand muscles with normal lower extremity strength. Muscle stretch reflexes were brisk with bilateral, sustained ankle clonus and bilateral extensor plantar responses. He walked with a spastic ataxic gait and could not tandem walk.

A brain MRI was found to be normal. A cervical spine MRI showed evidence of spondylosis, which was described by the local radiologist as only "mild to moderate." A thoracic spine MRI scan and CSF examination were normal.

He was diagnosed with presumed "transverse myelitis" related to bronchial infection.

A repeat cervical spine MRI was unchanged; however, the results were now reinterpreted to be evidence of advanced spinal stenosis at C4-C5 and C5-C6 levels with associated non-enhancing T2

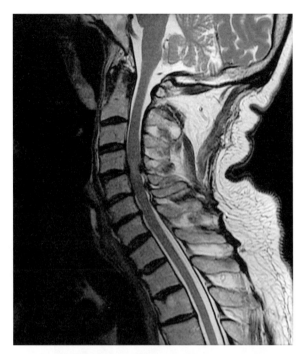

Figure 9.4 Sagittal T2 MRI cervical spine showing multilevel cervical spinal stenosis, advanced at C4-C5, with associated cord signal at this level compatible with spondylotic myelopathy.

hyperintensity within the cord, which are consistent with compressive spondylotic myelopathy (Figure 9.4).

Three-step assessment

1 Classical clinical features of MS: progressive myelopathy
2 Neurological examination: consistent with myelopathy
3 Investigations: MRI brain not consistent with MS; MRI cervical spinal cord consistent with compressive etiology; MRI thoracic spinal cord normal; CSF normal

Diagnosis: Compressive cervical spondylotic myelopathy.

Tip: Progression for more than four weeks is less compatible with inflammatory myelopathy such as transverse myelitis. Exclusion of compressive cervical spondylotic myelopathy is a critical initial step in evaluating and treating patients with myelopathy. This patient underwent immediate cervical spinal decompressive surgery and had marked improvement immediately after.

Case 61: Acute myelopathy while undergoing shoulder surgery. Is it transverse myelitis?

A 72-year-old woman underwent elective rotator cuff surgery. She was recovering from the surgery well and was not on any medications. It was thought that she may have been vaccinated for pneumococcus while hospitalized. Two weeks after the surgery, she awoke with significant chest pain. She was taken by the EMT providers back to the hospital after administering aspirin. Initially, she was discharged after no significant impairment was found. The next evening, she developed severe lower extremity paralysis which manifested in thoracic sensory level and bladder dysfunction with an inability to urinate. She was hospitalized and received three days of intravenous corticosteroids and oral corticosteroids for six days on a decreasing dose with minimal improvement.

She remained with ongoing urinary urgency, hesitancy and rare bowel incontinence. Her motor impairment improved over a number of months. She had no previous symptoms of MS attacks or CNS demyelination in the past and no progressive neurological impairment. She had a history of hypertension, hyperlipidemia and coronary artery disease. There was no family history of MS or other neurological disease. Her diagnosis was of inflammatory transverse myelitis possibly related to vaccination.

On undergoing a neurological examination months later, a motor examination of the face and upper extremities were found to be normal. Reflexes were reduced in the upper extremities, and plantar responses were flexor bilaterally. Her gait was cautious. Vibratory and joint position senses were normal in the hands and feet. There was reduced sensation to pinpricks and temperature that was greater in the left than right leg and the back and abdomen on both sides.

A brain MRI showed small vessel ischemic changes but no changes of demyelination. A cervical spine MRI was normal. A thoracic spinal cord MRI scan showed evidence of abnormal signal at T1 through T3 without gadolinium enhancement. A repeat thoracic spine MRI showed evidence of a focal non-enhancing T2 signal abnormality at the T2 level in the expected location of the anterior spinal artery (Figure 9.5). There were no abnormal flow voids, gadolinium enhancement or other evidence of

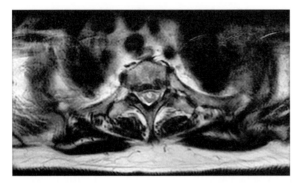

Figure 9.5 Axial T2 MRI thoracic spine shows a focal non-enhancing T2 hyperintensity along the ventral margin of the thoracic spinal cord at the T2 level in the expected location of the anterior spinal artery that is consistent with ischemic myelopathy.

an arteriovenous fistula. A lumbar spine MRI was normal. A CSF examination was normal, including the white blood cell count, IgG index and oligoclonal bands. West Nile Virus testing and NMO-IgG antibodies were both negative, as were an extensive battery of other viral and inflammatory markers on the serum and CSF. Chest and abdomen CTs were both normal.

Three-step assessment

Diagnosis: Ischemic thoracic myelopathy.

Tip: The morphology as well as the clinical presentation favored an ischemic myelopathy likely due to a small anterior spinal artery infarct rather than transverse myelitis. The acute onset with the severe pain, the MRI findings and the partial Brown-Sequard syndrome found on examination suggested an anterior spinal artery infarct as the cause rather than an inflammatory transverse myelitis. It was also confirmed later that the patient had not actually received any vaccination while in the hospital.

Case 62: A woman with left-sided pain and inflammatory myelopathy

A 51-year-old woman presented with an acute neurological event that had occurred six years previously following a routine influenza vaccination. At the time of the vaccination she developed a severe headache and facial pain that was possibly related to a sinus infection. She then developed significant fatigue and abdominal pain. On evaluation at a local emergency department she was found to have severe urinary retention requiring urinary catheterization. She then developed a painful band-like tightness involving the

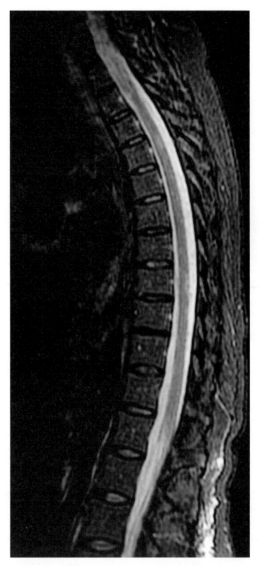

Figure 9.6 Sagittal T2 MRI thoracic spine shows subtle increased T2 signal within the thoracic spinal cord at the level of the T4 vertebral body extending less than one vertebral body height in length.

upper abdomen and lower chest. She was treated with intravenous methylprednisolone with "about 50 percent" improvement in the symptoms, with full improvement to normal after about one year aside from requiring gabapentin to control mild neuropathic pain. She had no recurrent symptoms or further symptoms of clinical attacks over the last six years.

On neurological examination, her mental status and cranial nerves were found to be normal. Her motor power and reflexes were normal with flexor plantar responses. A sensory examination and gait were normal.

Brain and cervical spine MRIs were normal. An initial thoracic spinal MRI demonstrated a single area of abnormal T2 (Figure 9.6), but a repeat thoracic spine MRI showed resolution of the area of abnormal signal. An initial CSF examination showed mild pleocytosis and mild elevation in the protein without unique CSF oligoclonal bands.

Three-step assessment

1 Classical clinical features of MS: acute myelopathy following vaccination without recurrence
2 Neurological examination: normal
3 Investigations: brain and cervical spine MRI normal; thoracic spinal cord MRIs consistent with prior inflammatory myelopathy with resolution; CSF normal

Diagnosis: Postvaccinal inflammatory thoracic myelitis with resolution.

Tip: When considering a diagnosis of postvaccinal myelitis, the onset of symptoms should come within only a few weeks after vaccination with no other clear cause being determined. Prolonged follow-up for new

inflammatory disease unrelated to vaccines or other inducing agents is important.

Case 63: A woman with progressive gait ataxia, myelopathy and peripheral neuropathy

A 48-year-old woman presented with gait disorder and peripheral neuropathy. Eight months prior to presentation, the patient developed tingling and loss of sensation in her feet, legs and hands. Over the following months, numbness and paresthesias increased in her legs and moved towards her waist. She had symptoms of sensory ataxia and had to watch herself while walking to prevent herself from falling.

On neurological examination, her cranial nerve examination was normal, while a motor examination revealed mild weakness in the intrinsic hand muscles bilaterally. Muscle stretch reflexes were increased with clonus and plantar responses were extensor bilaterally. She had loss of sensation to joint position sense, vibration, pinprick and light touch. She also had a wide-based, spastic, ataxic gait and a Romberg test was positive.

A brain MRI showed no significant abnormality. A cervical spine MRI showed T2 signal abnormality at

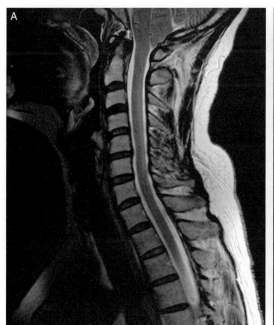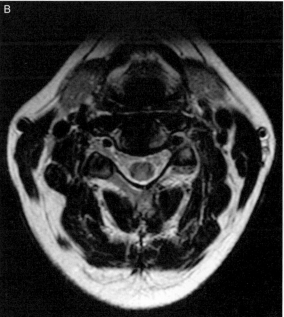

Figure 9.7 Sagittal and axial T2 MRI cervical spine showing T2 signal abnormality at the paramedian dorsal cervical cord, spanning the interval between C2–3 and C7, most evident at superior cord levels.

the paramedian dorsal cervical cord spanning C2 through C7, which was most evident at the superior cord levels without gadolinium enhancement or mass effect (Figure 9.7). A CSF examination was normal apart from a mild elevation of protein at 75 mg/dL. An electromyography (EMG) showed moderate length-dependent primarily axonal peripheral neuropathy. Serological testing showed normal values for vitamin B12, folate, intrinsic factor antibody, arylsulfatase A, hexosaminidase levels, vitamin E, paraneoplastic screen, syphilis serology, lyme serology, hepatitis screen, methylmalonic acid, very long-chain fatty acids, serum lactate and a peripheral smear for acanthocytes. Her ceruloplasmin level was reduced at 1.6 mg/dL (normal range 15 mg/dL −30 mg/dL). Her serum copper levels were markedly reduced at 0.11 mcg/mL (normal range 0.75 mcg/mL 1.45 mcg/mL).

Three-step assessment

1 Classical clinical features of MS: progressive myelopathy
2 Neurological examination: consistent with myelopathy
3 Investigations: brain MRI not suggestive of MS; cervical spinal cord – dorsal column predominance; CSF – no evidence of MS, non-specific elevation in protein; EMG – axonal peripheral neuropathy; serology – copper deficiency

   Diagnosis: Copper deficient myeloneuropathy.

   Tip: The presentation of the myeloneuropathy is highly consistent with copper deficiency myeloneuropathy as the cause. This mimics a longitudinal extensive myelitis such as neuromyelitis optica, but the distribution in the posterior part of the cord is most similar to that of subacute combined degeneration of the cord seen with vitamin B12 deficiency.

Case 64: A man with a longitudinal spinal cord lesion and pain. Is it a spinal cord neoplasm?

A 52-year-old right-handed man with a long history of low back and neck pain with numerous cervical and lumbar region surgeries was evaluated for intrascapular back pain. He had developed lower extremity weakness with numbness in the left leg to the lower thigh. The right leg was numb to the knee.

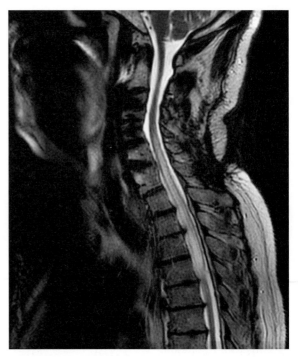

Figure 9.8 Sagittal T2 MRI cervical and thoracic spine shows T2 signal hyperintensity and cord expansion extending from approximately C5 to T5. Cord expansion is greatest at the T3 and T4 levels. Multilevel degenerative disc disease includes a large right paracentral disc protrusion at T2–T3.

On neurological examination, his cranial nerves, upper extremity and facial sensation were normal. He had mild motor weakness of the hamstrings, tibialis anterior and bilateral toe extensors. Reflexes were reduced in the upper and lower extremities, and his plantar responses were mute bilaterally. His vibratory sense was impaired to the ankle on the left and the mid-tibia knee on the right.

A brain MRI scan was normal. A spine MRI showed evidence of disc disease with an area of abnormal signal within the central thoracic cord (Figure 9.8). His CSF protein was elevated at 95 mg/dL but the CSF IgG index, oligoclonal bands, NMO-IgG and paraneoplastic autoantibody screen were all negative or normal.

A neurosurgical evaluation determined that the thoracic cord had herniated through the dura. Decompressive surgery was performed, which markedly improved his symptoms. A spinal cord biopsy at the same time showed no evidence of intraspinal neoplasm or an alternative cause.

Three-step assessment

1 Classical clinical features of MS: subacute myelopathy
2 Neurological examination: consistent with myelopathy
3 Investigations: brain MRI not suggestive of MS; thoracic spinal cord – disc disease and spinal cord dural herniation; spinal cord biopsy – no neoplastic or demyelinating disease

Diagnosis: Myelopathy due to dural thoracic spinal cord herniation.

Tip: Dural spinal cord herniations may present with a progressively worsening thoracic myelopathy. This etiology of a progressive myelopathy is uncommon. A spinal cord MRI may show a longitudinal T2 lesion and the evidence of the dural herniation may be difficult to appreciate. A neurosurgical evaluation is required to release and repair the herniation.

Case 65: An elderly woman with progressive lower extremity weakness and longitudinal thoracic spinal cord abnormality

An 80-year-old woman presented with a three-month history of lower extremity weakness. She had progressively worsening pain radiating from the right buttock into the right leg and started to use a walker for ambulation. Four months later she had worsening numbness in the lower extremities.

On examination, she had lower extremity weakness, proximally more than distally, in an upper motor neuron pattern. Her reflexes were increased, but she had absent ankle jerks. Her plantar responses were extensor bilaterally.

A brain MRI was normal. An initial thoracic spine MRI showed abnormal T2 signal in the central cord from the T5 vertebral level into the conus medullaris; there was also patchy intrinsic gadolinium enhancement within the thoracic cord. A repeat thoracic MRI four months later, however, showed extensive abnormal T2 signal in the thoracic cord with cord expansion and abnormal gadolinium enhancement on the ventral aspect from T8 through L1 (Figure 9.9). An MR angiogram of the spinal cord showed no convincing evidence of any abnormal vascularity in the spinal canal. A spinal angiography identified spinal epidural fistula located on the left at L2 (Figure 9.10). There was evidence of filling of an epidural venous pouch

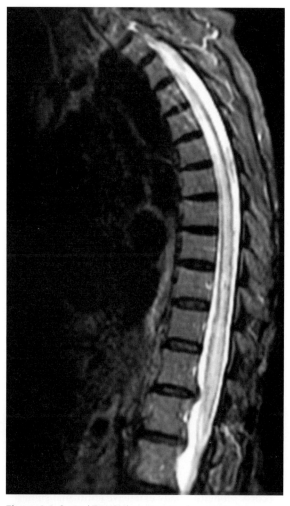

Figure 9.9 Sagittal T2 MRI thoracic spine shows extensive abnormal patchy T2 hyperintensity in cord with mild associated cord expansion, T4–L1.

adjacent to the left L2 pedicle. The pouch then drained into a vein which entered the dura and coursed superiorly. A CSF examination showed one white blood cell, very elevated protein at 111 mg/dL with a normal CSF IgG index and no unique CSF oligoclonal bands, while a cytology was negative for malignancy. Her serum neuromyelitis optica (NMO) aquaporin-4 levels as well as the angiotensin-converting enzyme (ACE) level were negative.

Three-step assessment

1 Classical clinical features of MS: progressive myelopathy
2 Neurological examination: consistent with myelopathy

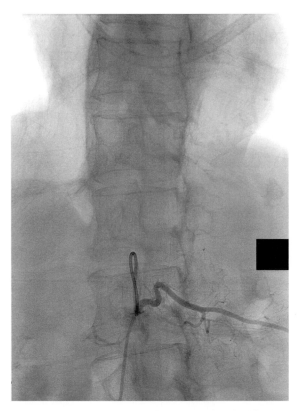

Figure 9.10 Spinal angiography showing spinal epidural fistula located on the left at L2. There was filling of an epidural venous pouch adjacent to the left L2 pedicle. The pouch then drains into a vein which enters the dura and courses superiorly.

3 Investigations: brain MRI normal; thoracic spinal cord – longitudinally extensive abnormal signal into conus medullaris; spinal angiogram – dural arteriovenous fistula identified

  Diagnosis: Spinal dural arteriovenous malformation.

  Tip: Spinal dural arteriovenous fistulas commonly present as progressive myelopathies that worsen over many months. A direct communication exists between the arterial and venous vasculature that produces increasingly high pressure and subsequent venous congestion with a risk of spinal cord ischemia. Men are affected more commonly than women and the thoracic spinal cord is more affected than the cervical cord. MRI features include high T2 signal extending distally into the conus, often with serpiginous dilatation of the venous plexus on the dorsal surface of the spinal cord. Prompt diagnosis is crucial to guide surgical or endovascular disconnection of the fistula.

Further reading

Atkinson JL, Miller GM, Krauss WE, et al. Clinical and radiographic features of dural arteriovenous fistula, a treatable cause of myelopathy. *Mayo Clin Proc* 2001;**76**: 1120–30.

Schmalstieg WF, Keegan BM, Weinshenker BG. Solitary sclerosis: progressive myelopathy from solitary demyelinating lesion. *Neurology* 2012;**78**:540–4.

Flanagan EP, Krecke KN, Marsh RW, Giannini C, Keegan BM, Weinshenker BG. Specific pattern of gadolinium enhancement in spondylotic myelopathy. *Ann Neurol* 2014;**76**:54–65.

Transverse Myelitis Consortium Working G. Proposed diagnostic criteria and nosology of acute transverse myelitis. *Neurology* 2002;**59**:499–505.

Scott TF, Frohman EM, De Seze J, Gronseth GS, Weinshenker BG. Evidence-based guideline: Clinical evaluation and treatment of transverse myelitis. *Neurology* 2011.

Berg-Johnsen J, Ilstad E, Kolstad F, Zuchner M, Sundseth J. Idiopathic ventral spinal cord herniation: an increasingly recognized cause of thoracic myelopathy. *J Cent Nerv Syst Dis* 2014;**6**:85–91.

Chhetri SK, Mills RJ, Shaunak S, Emsley HC. Copper deficiency. *BMJ* 2014;**348**:g3691.

De Souza RB, De Aguiar GB, Daniel JW, Veiga JC. The pathophysiology, classification, treatment, and prognosis of a spontaneous thoracic spinal cord herniation: A case study with literature review. *Surg Neurol Int* 2014;**5**:S564–6.

Frohman EM, Wingerchuk DM. Clinical practice. *Transverse myelitis. The New England Journal of Medicine* 2010;**363**:564–72.

Goodman BP. Metabolic and toxic causes of myelopathy. *Continuum* (Minneap Minn) 2015;**21**:84–99.

Hacein-Bey L, Konstas AA, Pile-Spellman J. Natural history, current concepts, classification, factors impacting endovascular therapy, and pathophysiology of cerebral and spinal dural arteriovenous fistulas. *Clin Neurol Neurosurg* 2014;**121**:64–75.

Karadimas SK, Gatzounis G, Fehlings MG. Pathobiology of cervical spondylotic myelopathy. *Eur Spine J* 2015;**24** Suppl 2:132–8.

Kumar N. Metabolic and toxic myelopathies. *Semin Neurol* 2012;**32**:123–36.

Marcus J, Schwarz J, Singh IP, et al. Spinal dural arteriovenous fistulas: a review. *Curr Atheroscler Rep* 2013;**15**:335.

Nouri A, Tetreault L, Singh A, Karadimas SK, Fehlings MG. Degenerative Cervical Myelopathy:

Epidemiology, Genetics and Pathogenesis. *Spine* (Phila Pa 1976) 2015.

Porrino J, Scherer KF, Gellhorn A, Avellino AM. Dural herniation of the spinal cord: a rare cause of myelopathy with unique imaging features. *PM R* 2014;**6**:1063–5.

Rubin MN, Rabinstein AA. Vascular diseases of the spinal cord. *Neurol Clin* 2013;**31**:153–81.

Vargas MI, Gariani J, Sztajzel R, et al. Spinal Cord Ischemia: Practical Imaging Tips, Pearls, and Pitfalls. *AJNR Am J Neuroradiol* 2014.

Index